T0220998

Disputes in Bioethics

NOTRE DAME STUDIES IN MEDICAL ETHICS

AND BIOETHICS

O. Carter Snead, series editor

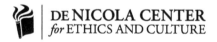

The purpose of the Notre Dame Studies in Medical Ethics and Bioethics series, sponsored by the de Nicola Center for Ethics and Culture, is to publish works that explore the ethical, cultural, and public questions arising from advances in biomedical technology, the practice of medicine, and the biosciences.

DISPUTES

in

BIOETHICS

Abortion, Euthanasia, and Other Controversies

CHRISTOPHER KACZOR

University of Notre Dame Press

Notre Dame, Indiana

University of Notre Dame Press
Notre Dame, Indiana 46556
undpress.nd.edu
All Rights Reserved

Copyright © 2020 by the University of Notre Dame

Published in the United States of America

Library of Congress Control Number: 2020940883

ISBN 978-0-268-10809-0 (Hardback)
ISBN 978-0-268-10810-6 (Paperback)
ISBN 978-0-268-10812-0 (WebPDF)
ISBN 978-0-268-10811-3 (Epub)

For Jennifer,

amo te

Contents

Prologue   ix

One   Is Speciesism a Form of Prejudice?   1

Two   What Is Dignity?   11

Three   Should We Make Children with Three (or More) Parents?   19

Four   Is *Roe v. Wade* Unquestionably Correct?   27

Five   What Are Reproductive Rights?   43

Six   Is It Better Never to Have Been Born?   53

Seven   Is There a Right to the Death of the Fetus?   61

Eight   Why Should the Baby Live?   71

Nine   Do Children Have a Right to Be Loved?   93

Ten   Do Children Contribute to the Flourishing of Their Parents?   101

Eleven   Is "Death with Dignity" a Dangerous Euphemism?   119

Twelve   Should Euthanasia Be Permitted for Children?   135

Thirteen   Does Assisted Suicide Harm Those Who Do Not Choose to Die?   143

Fourteen Is Conscientious Objection to Abortion Like 153
Conscientious Objection to Antibiotics?

Fifteen Do Medical Conscientious Objectors Differ from 161
Military Conscientious Objectors?

Sixteen Should Conscientiously Objecting Institutions Cover 169
Elective Abortion in Their Insurance Plans?

Seventeen Is It Ethically Permissible to Separate Conjoined Twins? 177

Acknowledgments 191

Notes 193
Bibliography 213
Index 223

Prologue

Disputes in Bioethics: Abortion, Euthanasia, and Other Controversies examines some of the central issues in contemporary bioethics. This collection of essays takes up questions about the dawn of human life, including "Should We Make Children with Three (or More) Parents?," "Is It Better Never to Have Been Born?," and "Why Should the Baby Live?" This volume also asks about the dusk of human life: "Is 'Death with Dignity' a Dangerous Euphemism?," "Should Euthanasia Be Permitted for Children?," and "Does Assisted Suicide Harm Those Who Do Not Choose to Die?" Still other questions are asked concerning recent views that health care professionals should not have a right to conscientiously object to legal and accepted medical practices. While we may accept conscientious objection to military service, recent scholars have argued that we should not accept conscientious objection to providing medical services because of important differences between the cases of medical and military objection. Another scholar has recently argued that conscientious objection to abortion makes no more sense than conscientious objection to antibiotics. Finally, the book also addresses questions about separating conjoined twins as well as the issue of whether the species of an individual makes a difference for the individual's moral status.

Eschewing the dominant perspectives of consequentialism and principalism, *Disputes in Bioethics* addresses recent and influential perspectives in contemporary bioethics from a methodology that maintains the inherent dignity of all human beings, who (it is argued) merit protection of their basic human goods. As an approach to bioethics, I work within the natural law tradition. I only tangentially address in this book rival

approaches such as utilitarianism or principalism. I view these rival frameworks as less compelling than natural law tradition and suggest that readers interested in my approach consult works, such as Alasdair MacIntyre's
Three Rival Versions of Moral Inquiry, that examine the natural law tradition in conversation with competing ethical theories. I am also, in this
book, not adjudicating among various versions of natural law, such as new
natural law (represented by figures such as Germain Grisez, John Finnis,
and Robert George) and classic natural law (represented by figures such as
Ralph McInerny, Russell Hittinger, and Stephen Brock). Likewise, I could
have included a chapter that engages rival frameworks in recent Catholic
moral theology. My book *Proportionalism and the Natural Law Tradition*
focuses on the latter and touches also on the former. Rather than retrace
this ground, I refer readers in notes to other sources that address such issues in greater depth.

The topics discussed in this work are of interest to readers both inside
and outside the academy. I hope it contributes to the ongoing discussion
of issues of signal importance. Finally, I would like to thank for support
in writing parts of this book the James Madison Program of Princeton
University.

One

Is Speciesism a Form of Prejudice?

WHAT IS THE MORAL STATUS OF NONRATIONAL ANIMALS? IS IT A SIN, comparable to racism or sexism, to treat your own species as superior to other species? What, if anything, makes the human person worthy of a special respect? Questions such as these form the contemporary discussion of animal rights, a topic of ongoing interest for applied ethics.

In a lecture delivered at the 2015 Society for Applied Philosophy Annual Conference, Shelly Kagan makes an important contribution to these debates. He takes aim at Peter Singer's proposition that "speciesism . . . is a prejudice or attitude of bias in favor of the interests of members of one's own species and against those of members of other species."[1] Racism is a prejudice or attitude of bias in favor of the interests of members of one's own race and against those of members of other races. Sexism is a prejudice or attitude of bias in favor of the interests of members of one's own sex and against those of members of the opposite sex. So too, according to Singer, speciesism is a moral mistake.

Initially subscribing to these views in the mid-1970s, Kagan has now become skeptical of the wrongfulness of speciesism. He thinks that our treatment of animals is generally unjustifiable and wrong but also holds that speciesism is not a mere prejudice because the interests of human beings count more than the interests of nonrational animals. Why? Kagan holds that all human beings are at least modal persons, individuals who could have been persons in the Lockean sense of "person." This modal property gives individual human beings a higher moral status, other things being equal, than animals.

Kagan notes that virtually no one holds that only the interests of human beings count or that the interests of animals are irrelevant. No one thinks that setting fire to a cat without any reason whatsoever is permissible. Nor does anyone hold that any trivial human interest outweighs every animal interest. The human desire to find out what a burning cat sounds like wouldn't justify dousing Mittens with gasoline and lighting a match. A more plausible view is that human interests count, in some yet unspecified way, as more important than animal interests. Implicit in the entire analysis is the assumption of consequentialism, shared by Kagan and Singer, which maintains that ethics is about maximizing interests, welfare, et cetera.

"What exactly is supposed to be wrong with speciesism?" asks Kagan.[2] The answer, according to Singer, is that it violates the principle of equal consideration of interests. To give greater weight to those of one's own race, or to those of one's own sex, or to those of one's own species, is to act arbitrarily and unfairly. If we wouldn't allow a human infant or mentally handicapped adult to be subject to medical experimentation for the sake of others, we should not subject animals, of equal or greater cognitive capacity, to the same sort of experiments. Pain is pain, whether suffered by an animal or by a human being.

This claim might be challenged in various ways. Death is death, whether suffered by a human being or by an animal. But Singer himself views the ethics of killing competent adult humans differently than that of killing nonhuman animals. By parity of reasoning, there may also be important ways that the pain of animals differs from the pain of human beings such that it is a mistake to assume that all that matters in the assessment of pain is its intensity and its duration. Moreover, certain kinds of suffering—like despair over failed life plans—cannot be experienced (as far as we know) by nonhuman animals.

Is speciesism a prejudice? It could be if it were based on false empirical beliefs, such as the erroneous opinion that animals feel no pain. But Kagan says an ethical prioritizing of human beings over animals could also be based on something else: "If one's speciesism is based instead on a direct appeal to moral intuition—and that is how I envision the speciesist—and if one is then prepared to give presumptive weight to moral intuitions in other matters as well, then that, it seems to me, is not prejudice. The view in question may or may not be correct; but it is not a mere prejudice and nothing more. So Singer's argument against speciesism fails."[3]

In 1776, the American Founders asserted that it was a self-evident truth that all human beings are created equal and endowed with inalienable rights. (Although some interpreters claim that the founders included only landowning, white men, I believe this interpretation is mistaken.) This proposition is a postulate of the Declaration of Independence that is not justified by still prior premises. Every argument must ultimately depend on some first principles that are not demonstrated on the basis of some prior suppositions. Singer, too, must rely on the intuition of first principles at various points in his argument.

Kagan goes on to point out that very few people are absolute speciesists at all. Imagine a scenario in which the evil Lex Luthor, wielding weapons of kryptonite, attacks the innocent Superman. We would, presumably, have the intuition that Luthor wrongs Superman in attacking him. Kagan writes, "Superman isn't human. He isn't a member of our biological species. But is there anyone (other than Lex Luthor!) who thinks this makes a difference? Is there anyone who thinks: Superman isn't human, so his interests should count less than they would if he were? I doubt it."[4] Indeed, many people of faith explicitly reject the idea that human beings and human beings alone have moral status as persons. For example, Christians believe in a Trinity of Divine Persons, angelic persons, and demonic persons. It is not being *human* that is necessary for being a person, but being an individual substance of a rational nature. So, following Kagan, Christians might say they are not speciesists but personists. What is necessary is not that the individual shares our species but that the individual is a person.

Kagan writes that "it is conceivable that being a person is not an all or nothing affair—but rather something that comes in degrees. Perhaps then a personist should be prepared to allow that the special consideration that comes with being a person can itself come in degrees as well."[5] Kagan does not address this issue at length, but we can explore it further. One way to approach the issue is to consider the question, how are persons to be treated? Thomas Aquinas held that we should imitate God and that God relates to persons (beings with a rational nature) "as objects of care for their own sakes; while other creatures are subordinated, as it were, to the rational creatures."[6] A Kantian might say persons are beings who deserve to be treated as ends in themselves rather than used simply as means.[7] A contemporary philosopher might add that the goods of persons give us ultimate reasons for action rather than merely instrumental ones.[8]

These views about the treatment due to persons suggest that "person" is a binary concept rather than a scalar one. In other words, an individual either is or is not a person. There is no scale of persons, from greater to lesser, but rather an equality of persons. To be a person is to merit treatment for one's own sake as an end, to be worthy of respect, not mere use, and to be an ultimate reason for action. Instrumental reasons can come in degrees as the usefulness of things comes in degrees. Something may be a more or less effective means to some end. A hammer is a more effective means of driving nails and a less effective means of driving screws in comparison to the screwdriver. By contrast, someone, a person, is in a radically different category. She is an individual to be cared for, an end in herself, an ultimate reason for action. The binary nature of personhood undergirds the equality of persons, since individuals who are persons are all equally ends in themselves and ultimate reasons for action.

Are there any nontheological grounds for the view that human beings should be accorded a greater moral status than animals? Thomas Aquinas claims that we should love the greater good more than the lesser good. Thus we should love a virtuous person more than a vicious person. Of course, since all persons are fundamentally equal, they are all due a fundamental respect. But we can go beyond fundamental respect by, for example, appreciating the distinctive goods of particular persons.

The view that personhood is nonscalar (either an individual is an end in herself or not an end in herself, either an individual has basic rights or does not) is fully compatible with Thomas's idea that we should love virtuous people more than we love vicious people. Thomas's view is that all human beings deserve to be treated as persons. So, for example, to treat a person as if she were an inanimate object would be an injustice. There is a fundamental baseline of respectful treatment that all persons deserve. At the same time, if we think of love as partially involving appreciation of the goodness of the beloved, and if there is more goodness in a virtuous person than in a vicious person, then there is more to appreciate in a virtuous person than in a vicious person. In terms of appreciation, therefore, it is appropriate to have a deeper love for virtuous persons than for vicious persons. Of course, for Thomas, other factors are also relevant for the kind of love that is fitting for an individual. For example, the proximity of relationship is also a factor for determining how much love is appropriate for an individual.[9] Other things being equal, I should love my own mother more than other mothers. And so, it could turn out, I should love my mother more than others even if she is less virtuous than others. But I should treat all mothers, indeed all human beings, with a fundamental respect, even if my love for human beings is unequal.

In terms of goodness of nature, however, all human beings share a nature that is greater in goodness than the nature of animals like dogs. And what is meant here by nature? Thomas writes, "We call the nature of each thing that which belongs to it when its generation is perfect; for example, the nature of man is that which he possesses once his generation is perfect."[10] Thomas is making the point that the nature of a thing is manifest in the perfected generation of the thing, whether the thing in question is a horse or a human. A fully mature and healthy human being enjoys perfections such as rational speech, friendship, and understanding of abstract truths that are not enjoyed by the fully mature and healthy horse. Both the horse and the human can enjoy goods such as health, but the human can also enjoy goods such as knowing the truth about God. In this way, human nature is oriented to greater goods than horse nature, so in this sense to be a human is a greater thing than to be a horse. If we should love greater things more than lesser things, then we have reason to love every human being more than any horse, at least with respect to their different natures.

Both human beings and nonrational animals alike have sentient natures; they exist, live, and sense. Human beings alone, as far as we know of creatures on earth, also have a rational nature. Their perfection is found in goods such as understanding and living in accordance with the truth, living with personal integrity, and forming friendships of virtue. Thus human nature is greater in goodness than animal nature, having everything contained in animal nature and more. Because of the greater goodness of their nature, human beings should be loved more than animals.

The view that human beings should be accorded a greater moral status than animals therefore differs radically from both sexism and racism. Human nature, as rational, contains greater goodness than mere sentient nature or vegetative nature, so individuals with a human nature should be loved more than beings with only a sentient or vegetative nature. Similarly, Aquinas holds that individual persons with divine nature—Father, Son, and Holy Spirit—should be loved more than individuals with human nature by virtue of the greater goodness of divine nature in comparison to human nature. Since male and female human beings share equally in human nature, they are equally to be loved in that respect. In a similar way, the various races of human beings all share in the same human nature, so they too are to be equally loved. So there is no inconsistency in defending the greater dignity of humans above animals but condemning sexism or racism. Equality in nature provides grounds both for supporting ethical humanism and for condemning prejudice.

Does holding that all human beings have basic rights imply a bias in favor of one's own species? Not at all. I believe that I am a human being, but let's say I am wrong. Suppose I merely appear to be human, but it turns out that I am actually of the same species as Superman, who looks, sounds, and usually acts like a human being but is really a Kryptonian. Let's say that today I discover my superpowers and realize that I, too, am a Kryptonian. If I realized I was not human, I would still hold that human beings have a higher moral status than all animals lacking a rational nature. I would also realize that there are other beings that have a rational nature, namely, Kryptonians. The question of whether human beings belong to my own species is therefore irrelevant for defending the view that all human beings have intrinsic dignity and basic rights.

In his *Grounding for the Metaphysics of Morals*, Immanuel Kant articulated this fundamental principle of ethics: "Act in such a way that you treat humanity, whether in your own person or in the person of another, always at the same time as an end and never simply as a means."[11] Note that Kant does not say that *only* humanity, whether ourselves or others, is to be treated as ends and never used as means. Kant's principle is open to the possibility that other species should also be treated as ends in themselves and never used simply as means. Maybe there are other species such as Kryptonians or angels who merit this respect, or maybe humanity is the only such species. Kant leaves these as open questions. Also left open is the possibility that some other characteristic, such as sentience, is sufficient for moral status. Kant's principle, as stated, is strictly neutral with respect to this possibility. It claims only that humanity deserves respect, not that *only* humanity deserves respect. If someone says that all women deserve respect, that person is not even implicitly denying that men and children also deserve respect. Kant's view stands in opposition to the claim that species is irrelevant for moral status (thus standing in tension with Singer's position), but it leaves open the possibility that other species may also have moral status (in this respect compatible with Singer's position).

In his article "Modal Personhood and Moral Status," David DeGrazia assumes with Kagan that human beings who are not and never will function rationally are not persons. "If a human being is not a person but would have been if not for some improbable accident that occurred when he was an infant, we may rationally regret his lack of personhood. But it is much less clear that the fact that he could have been a person constitutes a reason to regard him as having higher moral status than he enjoys just on the basis of his categorical (as opposed to modal) properties."[12] DeGrazia recognizes a key element in Kagan's view. There is something lamentable, a rational regret, in a human being who is not able to exercise his or her rational nature, but there is nothing regrettable in a dog not being able to exercise rational nature because the dog lacks a rational nature.

Suppose that we discover a medical intervention that enables both a dog and a brain-damaged human being to function rationally. Would our decision to give the treatment either to the dog or to the human being really be a matter of moral indifference? A dog can live a full and flourishing canine life without ever functioning rationally. Indeed, a functionally rational dog might well be miserable because it would be cut off from the canine community and also socially isolated from humans. By contrast, a human being does not have a canine life to fall back on if she cannot function rationally. The nature of the individual in question is relevant for determining what interventions should be given. Since all human beings have a rational nature, interventions that enable rational functioning restore health. Since the nature of a human differs from the nature of a dog, the flourishing of the human person differs from the flourishing of a dog. As Aristotle noted, rationality plays a constitutive role in human flourishing, so a lack of ability to function rationally constitutes a grave disability for a (mature) human being but not for a mature dog.

The enhanced-dog example is sometimes used to argue against the view of personhood as endowment. If we could enhance the intelligence of Fido just a little bit each day, say by an injection that permanently boosts intelligence two IQ points, eventually the dog would be as intelligent as you or me. Enhanced-Fido would be as much a person as Benjamin Franklin. The enhanced-dog example shows, so it is argued, that endowment, nature, and species are irrelevant to moral status, since Fido remains numerically the same canine in these respects before, during, and after the injections.[13]

One way to approach the enhanced-dog example is to say that small accidental changes sometimes lead to a substantial change. If my blood pressure gradually drops, at some point just a small drop further will cause it to crash and my life to end. A tiny subtraction can lead to the substantial change from life to death. The enhanced-dog example could be understood as a gradual enhancement that causes a substantial change, which transforms a nonrational animal into a rational animal. Another possibility is that the enhanced-dog example teaches us to understand something about dogs that we never understood before. We always assumed, on the basis of empirical observation, that the only animals who could function rationally were human beings, so human beings were the only animals with a rational nature. But if it turned out that other animals could, through training or medical enhancement, also function rationally, then they too would be rational animals. Our assumptions about the kinds of activities individuals or things do to reveal what sort of natures they have are always open to correction. But I seriously doubt such corrections will actually happen, so ethically speaking we have no need to revise our working assumption that only human beings are rational animals.

In "Why Speciesism Is Wrong: A Response to Kagan," Singer says the capacity to suffer is both the sufficient and necessary condition for an individual to have moral status:

> If a being suffers there can be no moral justification for refusing to take that suffering into consideration. No matter what the nature of

the being, the principle of equality requires that its suffering be counted equally with the like suffering—insofar as rough comparisons can be made—of any other being. If a being is not capable of suffering, there is nothing to be taken into account. So the limit of sentience (using the term as a convenient if not strictly accurate shorthand for the capacity to suffer and/or experience enjoyment) is the only defensible boundary of concern for the interests of others.[14]

The capacity to suffer is the only defensible boundary if we presuppose that suffering alone counts in coming to moral judgments. But why should we think that suffering *alone* counts in our moral judgments of what is right and what is wrong? Let us say that students blacken your reputation by claiming that you are an unfair teacher who harasses them, but you never learn of their calumny. Indeed, no one believes their charges, so your reputation with your colleagues does not change at all. So no suffering whatsoever occurs. Did the students do something wrong in lying about you and trying to ruin your reputation? If so, then more than suffering is at stake in coming to our moral judgment, since in this case no one suffered. Let's say that at your funeral, colleagues spread lies about you to damage your reputation: have they not done something wrong? Presumably, you won't suffer on account of their lies. Unless we are utilitarians supposing that only suffering and enjoyment ultimately matter, why should we think that moral status necessarily depends on the capacity for suffering and enjoyment?

Singer continues, "I don't think plants have interests, in the morally relevant sense, any more than, say, a car guided through traffic by a computer would have an interest in reaching its destination. Neither plants nor the car are conscious. To imagine what it is like to be a pig in a factory farm is an idea that makes sense, even if it is difficult to get it right. Imagining yourself as a plant or a computer-guided car yields only a blank."[15] The supposition is that an individual needs to be conscious in order to have interests. But beings who are not conscious clearly do have interests. Imagining yourself as an unconscious person in surgery yields only a blank, but if you were in that situation, you would still have interests—not getting murdered, for example.

Is it wrong to take species into account when considering the moral status of an individual? This fascinating question has been given new impetus by the contributions of Kagan, DeGrazia, and Singer. Inasmuch as moral status has something to do with nature, and nature has something to do with species, there is nothing illegitimate in taking species into account when making moral judgments, including judgments about who has dignity.

Two

What Is Dignity?

DISCUSSIONS ABOUT DIGNITY CONTINUE UNABATED. WHAT DOES *DIGNITY* mean in the context of bioethics? Is dignity useless or useful? Can we reduce dignity to autonomy? For some authors, the ambiguity of dignity is part of the strength of this ethical concept. For example, Glenn Hughes suggests that an "intrinsically heuristic concept means that [the concept] refers to an intelligible reality of which we have some understanding, but whose full or complete content remains, and will always remain to some degree, unknown to us."[1] Dignity is a heuristic concept that can never be fully known, in part because the human person is ultimately a mystery.

Because we have some understanding of who we are individually and as human beings, the concept of human dignity is not without content. But just as we never fully understand ourselves or other human beings, we also never fully understand human dignity.

This line of thinking can be theologically developed. If we are made in God's image and likeness, then we must always remain at least somewhat unable to be fully comprehended. In the *Summa contra gentiles* and elsewhere, St. Thomas Aquinas taught that God cannot be fully comprehended. In this life, we cannot fully comprehend God because our understanding of who God is comes from the effects that God brings into being.

These effects allow us to partially but never fully understand the First Cause. But even in the life to come, the blessed in heaven do not fully comprehend God, because only an infinite Intellect can comprehend the Infinite Being of God. Even in heaven, only a Divine Mind can understand perfectly the Divine Being. Of course, it does not follow from this that the blessed in heaven or the faithful on earth can know nothing about God. However, the practice of apophatic or negative theology reminds us of the fragility of our knowledge of God.

If our knowledge of God is incomplete, fragile, and subject to development, then so too our knowledge of the human person made in God's image must be incomplete, fragile, and subject to development. Human dignity necessarily involves the human person, so our understanding of human dignity never reaches perfection as well.

In his article "Should Inherent Human Dignity Be Considered Intrinsically Heuristic?," Bharat Ranganathan argues that this ambiguity causes serious problems for dignity as a bulwark for human rights.[2] To the degree that a particular theological or metaphysical basis is given for human dignity, consensus for human dignity and therefore human rights is eroded. Moreover, if we cannot disambiguate human dignity, then we cannot use it to disambiguate various possible human rights. Ranganathan's concerns are well placed. It may be that speaking about the theological basis for dignity undermines the usefulness of the concept when addressing particular audiences. A pluralistic, secular audience will be left unpersuaded by a grounding of dignity in any particular theological or metaphysical framework. This weakness, though, is shared by all particular outlooks and conceptions. A utilitarian approach leaves the Kantian cold, and the Kantian approach provokes Aristotelian rejection. The fact that a particular theological or metaphysical basis for dignity is not shared by everyone counts against it as much as against any other justification that is also not shared by everyone. Here, we can note an important difference between theological and metaphysical grounding of dignity. A theological basis may, in certain frameworks, depend upon faith in divine revelation. So the ultimate basis for the belief would transcend reason in a way that metaphysical beliefs arising from reason alone do not. In any case, it is wise to consider the audience to which one is speaking. As Aquinas notes in the *Summa contra gentiles*, in arguments with Christians, appeal can be made to the

New Testament. In arguments with Jewish believers, appeal can be made to the Hebrew scriptures. In arguments with nonbelievers, appeal can be made only to reason.

Ranganathan is ultimately right that dignity cannot serve as useful in contemporary debate unless it is disambiguated. Fortunately, this work of clarifying various senses of the term has been carefully done by Daniel Sulmasy. In his article "The Varieties of Human Dignity: A Logical and Conceptual Analysis," Sulmasy distinguishes three senses of *dignity*: intrinsic, attributed, and inflorescent.[3] Once he clarifies the distinctions between these senses and establishes the proper logical relationship among them, Sulmasy shows that the term is not hopelessly ambiguous and therefore is not useless in bioethical debates.

To say someone has intrinsic dignity is to claim that the person has worth, value, and stature simply in virtue of being human. This dignity cannot be lost but rather remains as long as the human being remains. Just as every single living human being has the biological quality of being a mammal, so too every single living human being has the ethical quality of intrinsic dignity. Intrinsic dignity does not rely on the choices of anyone but is something that remains whether or not someone is recognized to have it.

Attributed dignity is something that human beings confer on one another by choice. If Princeton grants an honorary doctorate to a benefactor, the university enhances the attributed dignity of the benefactor. On the other hand, a jailer might undermine the attributed dignity of his captives by feeding them only dogfood or forcing them to parade around naked.

Finally, what Sulmasy calls inflorescent dignity consists in the wellbeing and flourishing of the person in question. When human beings live lives in which they are accorded respect and enjoy good health, warm friendships, and the deepening of knowledge, they enjoy inflorescent dignity. Dignity as flourishing depends in part on choice but also in part on circumstances beyond the power of human choice.

None of these three uses of the word *dignity* is the correct usage, but each sense of the term may be properly used in different contexts and for different purposes. Yet the various senses of the term *dignity* on Sulmasy's view are logically and linguistically related, with the intrinsic sense being the prior sense of the term.

Sulmasy's thesis is that attributed and inflorescent dignity presupposes both logically and linguistically the intrinsic sense of dignity. His disambiguation of the term *dignity* is valuable, but the argument he gives for the thesis is overly complex, consisting of nine numbered considerations and many subdivisions.

If I have understood his arguments correctly, they might be briefly summarized in the following way. Attributed dignity presupposes intrinsic dignity because we attribute dignity only to beings that we have already picked out as having intrinsic value. Inflorescent dignity presupposes intrinsic dignity because if the being in question is ultimately unimportant (lacking intrinsic dignity), then its flourishing is likewise ultimately unimportant.

If this construal of Sulmasy's argument is correct, then I do not think it is a sound argument. Some philosophers deny that any human being has intrinsic dignity but think that dignity arises at some point in human development, such as at viability, sentience, or self-conscious desire to continue existing. These authors also are perfectly capable of performing acts that bestow attributed dignity on others. Similar examples could be provided to indicate that inflorescent dignity also does not depend upon intrinsic dignity.

I wish Sulmasy had spent greater time in this article explaining his justification for intrinsic dignity, and perhaps he does in other writings. He holds that intrinsic dignity arises because of the law-like generalizations, typical features, and natural history of natural kinds, but it is not entirely clear to me how these considerations establish the conclusion that all human beings have intrinsic dignity. Sulmasy writes, "There might be those who would claim that only a morally indefensible speciesist bias could lead one to make distinctions in value among living things based on the observation of a gradation in the intrinsic value of biological natural kinds by virtue of increasing phylogenetic complexity."[4]

Can there be gradations among things with intrinsic value? Sherif Girgis argues that personhood in the moral sense cannot be a matter of degree, because if you matter not just instrumentally but intrinsically, if your well-being counts as an ultimate reason for action, then there cannot really be degrees of its counting.[5] On this understanding of intrinsic value, intrinsic value provides an ultimate reason for action that need not be grounded in any further justification. But if we understand intrinsic value in this sense, then it is hard to see how there could be gradations in intrinsic value.

Perhaps both Sulmasy and Girgis would agree to the following. If something has intrinsic value, then to use it simply as a means is to make a moral mistake. It is to treat someone who should be respected as an end, having value in himself or herself, as if the person were merely a tool with instrumental value.

Immanuel Kant's formulation of respecting humanity as an end in itself articulates this moral principle by maintaining that we should act in such a way that we treat humanity, whether in our own person or in the person of another, always at the same time as an end and never simply as a means. When someone acts against this principle, treating things that are mere means as if these things were ends in themselves, the mistake is apparent.

Imagine someone who set up his whole life in order to worship a mallet. Honoring the hammer, celebrating the nail driver, and contemplating its fine craftsmanship were the source and summit of his life. First thought of the day? About the hammer. Last thought before bed? Hammer time. He sacrifices his own well-being and the well-being of other people all for the sake of the hammer. It is no less irrational to treat persons—ends in themselves—as if they were merely things. To act in either way is to confuse what is merely a means with what is an end.

Like Sulmasy, Carlo Leget also seeks to disambiguate *dignity*.[6] Leget proposes three definitions: (1) social position, (2) intrinsic quality, and (3) dignity as experience—a purely subjective notion that "rests entirely on what individuals say they feel."[7] He then critiques each definition. Much of his analysis is sound. For example, Leget correctly notes that the problem with dignity as experience is that people can have mistaken views of themselves, as when a dangerously thin girl thinks that she is fat. However, when Leget turns to critiquing intrinsic dignity, his analyses are less persuasive.

One problem with intrinsic dignity, in Leget's view, is that "intrinsic dignity . . . in Stoic, Christian and Kantian philosophy . . . was used to divide the world into those rational and nonrational beings. Obviously this clarity has a price to be paid by both human beings whose rationality is compromised and higher mammals who display forms of social and rational behavior that we are still trying to understand."[8]

These considerations do not in fact undermine the notion of intrinsic dignity. If human beings have intrinsic dignity, then human beings who are compromised in terms of the exercise of their rationality are not compromised in terms of their dignity. An intrinsic quality is a quality that cannot be lost so long as the being in question continues to exist. Having sides is intrinsic to being a triangle, so as long as a triangle exists, a being with sides exists. Higher mammals, such as dolphins or great apes, also do not pose a challenge to the notion of intrinsic dignity. Such beings may have intrinsic dignity or such beings may not have it. We can have a fruitful argument about such matters. The fact that there are marginal cases in which it is unclear whether the concept applies does nothing to undermine the concept. It is unclear, and we may never know whether at this instance we have an odd or an even number of hairs on our head, but this fact does not mean that the concepts of odd and even numbers are themselves fuzzy.

Leget continues his critique of intrinsic dignity:

> A second problem, put forward by those who advocate a strong emphasis on experienced dignity, is that the idea of intrinsic dignity can work as an intellectual prison that may deny the experiences of people. If I feel that because of a fatal disease my dignity as a human person is compromised to such a degree that I see the continuation of my life as a hell but I live in a cultural context that forbids the termination of my life because of my dignity as a human being, I may feel held captive in life against my own will.[9]

Advocates of intrinsic dignity can push back on this argument by noting that the fact that people have intrinsic dignity does not deny the experiences of people who feel they have lost their dignity as experienced. Because people have intrinsic dignity, it matters morally what happens to them. If a person feels degraded because of loss of control or other factors that make them feel subhuman, this matters precisely because they still have intrinsic dignity. If the person really no longer counted morally, then we would not concern ourselves with their feelings or their experience of losing their sense of dignity. Moreover, some people have accepted the idea of intrinsic dignity and have also believed that intentional killing is justified. As I argue later in this book, I am not sure these two ideas are ultimately compatible. The earliest advocates of intrinsic dignity, the Stoics, also did not oppose suicide. So there is at least a prima facie compatibility of the two notions.

Some authors have pointed to an inconsistency between championing autonomy on the one hand and undermining intrinsic dignity on the other. Colin Bird points out this connection in the thought of Alan Gewirth: "Every human agent must attribute worth to his purposes . . . [because he] regards his purposes as good according to whatever criteria enter into his purposes."[10] If an agent sees his or her goals as worthwhile, implicitly that agent is also affirming some sense of personal worth. The agent is the source of the action. If the action is valuable, the agent must also be valuable. Gewirth puts the points as follows: "They are *his* purposes, and they are worth attaining because *he* is worth sustaining and fulfilling, so that he has what for him is a justified sense of his own worth."[11] The conclusion is that the "generic purposiveness" of rational action, just as such, "underlies the ascription of inherent dignity to all agents" (including oneself).[12] Why should we respect autonomy? The autonomy of a person matters only if the person matters. So it is not, in the metaphysical and moral order, that autonomy gives rise to the dignity of persons but rather that the dignity of persons gives rise to the value of autonomy. But this suggests that efforts such as those of Mary Ann Warren, Michael Tooley, Alberto Giubilini, and Francesca Minerva to ground the value of the human being in the autonomy of the human being are getting things backward.

Leget continues his critique of intrinsic dignity as follows: "A third problem focusing on intrinsic dignity alone is that paradoxically it may contribute to cleaning the consciousness of people and abstaining from moral action when it is urgent. If the intrinsic dignity of people cannot be taken away it may become an excuse for not helping them in need, e.g. when they are considered to be far away and not part of our own culture. Whatever famine or poverty people may suffer, their dignity can never be taken away from them."[13]

This concern, I think, is also not such a problem. Intrinsic dignity cannot be lost, which means that whoever has it is the subject of moral rights and deserves to be treated in a way that accords with his or her moral status. But this means that the notion of intrinsic dignity is not an invitation to inaction in the moral realm. Rather, the intrinsic dignity of each human being provides a reason for action to benefit every human being. Suffering and poverty do not take away the intrinsic dignity of people, but suffering and poverty invite upright people to care about the poor and the suffering and therefore seek to relieve their plight.

Three

Should We Make Children with Three (or More) Parents?

HOW COULD TECHNOLOGY CHANGE PARENTHOOD IN THE TWENTY-first century? In vitro fertilization and surrogate motherhood in the twentieth century created the need to distinguish different senses of parenthood: genetic parenthood—one's own genetic material, sperm or egg, giving rise to a child; gestational parenthood—the bearing of a developing human being in utero; and social parenthood—the rearing of a child to adulthood. With the advent of cloning, an individual person could become a genetic parent not only without the help of another person but even without consent and without having sex. Theoretically, cloning can take cells from a toothbrush used by LeBron James at the Ritz-Carlton and from it make his identical, much younger twin. What other changes are on the horizon?

Scientists seek to create artificial gametes from any human cell. If successful, they could make sperm from Jennifer Anniston's hair, or ova from George Clooney's fingernail. Researchers have already created artificial gametes in mice from their skin cells and used these gametes to produce fertile offspring.[1] Similar transformations may be possible in human beings. Before science fiction becomes science fact, we might want to consider the ethical ramifications of such innovations.

For example: Is it fair to spend vast sums of money to benefit the small number of people who want to use artificial gametes? It seems that this money could be better used to provide basic health care for many people or to fund research for cures of deadly diseases such as cancer or AIDS.[2] Anyone who advocates an ethics of maximizing human well-being cannot consistently condone spending money on artificial gametes when innumerable people lack healthy food and clean water. Let us, however, lay these kinds of considerations aside.

Let us also, for the sake of argument, reserve some of our ethical concerns about in vitro fertilization in order to consider some of the ethical consequences that result from this new technology. What other ethical considerations does this new technology raise? To create artificial gametes so as to study and ultimately alleviate the causes of infertility is not morally problematic in itself. To use artificial gametes for the production of new human beings, however, raises weighty ethical issues. The trouble, in part, is that the first project leads almost ineluctably to the second: "If you want to understand, you have to create it. If you want to understand how good an egg [created artificially] is, you have to fertilise."[3] These embryonic human beings will be either killed in experimentation or brought to birth. Obviously, if all human beings deserve basic rights, then these killings are impermissible. But using artificial gametes to create a child for birth is not itself without serious problems.

Additional ethical concerns come to mind. People created by artificial gametes may very well have increased likelihood of mental and physical disabilities. Moreover, we simply do not know what the long-term effects of such experimentation might be. We do not even know what the short-term effects will be, though we might be able, through animal testing, to have a fairly good idea. Even if extensive tests were to be conducted on nonhuman animals first, experimentation on human beings without their consent will take place if artificial gametes are used for reproduction. Such experimentation wrongs these human beings even if it does not harm them.

One response to such concerns is to note that without artificial gametes some human beings simply would not exist.[4] The choice, for those who put forward this opinion, is not between such persons coming into existence through normal sexual intercourse and coming into existence via artificial gametes. The choice is between existing via artificial gametes or not existing at all. So long as the persons created prefer life over nonexistence, they have not been harmed or wronged even if their lives are much worse off than those of other human beings.[5] Indeed, the use of artificial gametes could be seen as experimentation for the benefit of the child brought into existence.

In coming into existence, a human being is neither benefited nor harmed, at least if *benefited* means being made "better off" than previously and *harmed* means being made "worse off" than previously. *Better off* and *worse off* are comparative terms. Unless we believe in something like pre-existing souls, prior to a human being's coming into existence there is no state of well-being to which we may compare the present condition. But a human being is wronged not just when made "worse off," which is impossible in the case we are considering, but also when someone does not have that to which he or she is entitled or that which human beings can reasonably expect.[6] If the use of artificial gametes leads to disability in the children created, these children will have been wronged in not receiving that to which they were entitled and could reasonably expect, namely a normal likelihood of health.

Anna Smajdor and Daniela Cutas note other ethical issues raised by artificial gametes.[7] When you shake hands, some stray cells are exchanged. Given the possibility of artificial gametes, these cells could be used to create sperm and eggs genetically like your sperm or eggs. In this way, you could become the genetic parent of a child without your knowledge or consent.

Innumerable people would love to have children genetically related to NFL quarterbacks, Grammy winners, or cover girl fashionistas. Given technological advances, genetic parenthood could be achieved with virtually anyone with whom one had the slightest contact. Smajdor and Cutas point out that laws in most countries currently view genetic parenthood as the key to deciding who is or is not the legal father of a child—with responsibility for child support payments.

In their article "Artificial Gametes and the Ethics of Unwitting Parenthood," Smajdor and Cutas take up two central questions: "First, if unwitting genetic parenthood is feasible, is it acceptable to impose finan-cial parental responsibility on the basis of genetic evidence alone? Second, are people harmed if—without their consent—children are born who are genetically related to them?"[8] In order to address these questions, they consider a range of actual cases in which parenthood is nonvoluntary. One case involves a divorced couple fighting over their IVF embryos. She wants to bring them to term; he does not want to bring them to term. In another case, a woman has sex with a semi-passed-out man and gets pregnant. We could add the case of statutory rape in which an eighth-grade boy, obvi-ously too young to legally consent to sex, impregnates a woman. Should the male in each of these cases be held financially and morally responsible for the child?

These cases are not all alike. The first case—a married couple fighting over IVF embryos—does not involve making someone a parent against his will. Assuming it is a typical case of IVF, the man donated sperm precisely in order to conceive human embryos. Once a human being is conceived, the man has fathered a child. He is already a genetic father. Ordinary dis-course reflects the idea that fatherhood begins prior to birth. Medical per-sonnel ask pregnant women, "Who is the father?" not "Who is going to be the father?" The question is asked in the present tense because the child in utero or in vitro has a father. Likewise, once conception takes place, the woman whose egg gave rise to the new human being is the genetic mother. If the embryo is inside a woman's body, she is also the gestational mother. Fights over IVF embryos are not about making someone a parent but about making someone take responsibility for being a genetic parent.

Is being a genetic parent sufficient for someone to have an ethical re-sponsibility for a child? Parenthood, at least in the genetic and gestational senses, can be nonvoluntary. A woman who finds herself pregnant by rape is a genetic and gestational mother. A man could also find himself nonvol-untarily a parent if he fathers a child without his consent (say, in sexual intercourse in which he is incapacitated in such a way that he cannot con-sent to sex or is too young to give legal and moral consent). Do such per-sons who became parents against their will have special responsibilities for their biological children?

Intuitions on this point may vary. On the one hand, the well-being of the child must be a concern. Vulnerable young children need support. In some cases, we have special ethical responsibilities for those who are related to us (such as parents or siblings) even though we did not choose to have these relationships. Fathers and mothers have special obligations to support their own children.

On the other hand, in the case of the sexual abuse of a minor who is male or with a man whose genetic material is used without his consent, it does seem unfair to force him to pay child support. No one would force a woman who was raped to pay child support to the rapist raising their biological child.

But is it not—by parity of reasoning—also unfair to force a woman to continue gestating the child in a case of rape? In this case, the mother alone can support her child until he or she is old enough to be born. In a similar way, if the involuntary biological father alone is the only one in the position to support his child until he or she is old enough to be cared for by others, then he too has an obligation to care for the child.

Here is another case raised by Smajdor and Cutas: "Let us suppose that a man—Peter—strongly believes the world is overpopulated and therefore chooses not to reproduce. Someone [Sally] collects Peter's discarded skin cells in order to produce gametes and have a child, without his knowledge or consent. Has Peter been harmed? And if so, what if any action is he justified in taking? Can he destroy the gametes, embryos or offspring that have been created without his consent?"[9]

If all human beings have equal basic rights, then there is a prima facie case to be made that Peter may not licitly destroy his offspring. Whether Peter's child is in the infant, fetal, or embryonic stage of human development is irrelevant. Could Peter destroy his gametes prior to the creation of another human being? On this question, it seems that the answer would be affirmative because he may prevent the unauthorized use of what is his, and his sperm are his.

Did Sally harm Peter in producing gametes from his cells in order to create his biological child? Peter is not physically harmed, since the cells Sally used were discarded and do not impede his physical well-being in any way. Sally might harm Peter psychologically if Peter suffers anxiety or trauma after learning that he has a son or daughter. However, if Sally successfully conceals the existence of Peter's child from him, Peter will not suffer psychological harm from her action. Although she did not harm him physically or psychologically, Sally wronged Peter inasmuch as she used parts from Peter's body in a morally significant way without his consent.

If it is wrong to use someone else's body or body parts without consent, does this give rise to Judith Jarvis Thomson's famous Violinist Analogy for abortion? Unplanned pregnancy, according to Thomson, is like waking up plugged into a famous violinist who needs to use your kidneys for nine months in order to survive.[10] It would be very nice to allow the violinist to remain plugged into you, but you are not doing anything wrong by unplugging yourself from the violinist. Abortion may be justified even if the human being in utero has a right to live because women have no obligation to keep the human fetus alive. In an unwanted pregnancy, the woman's body is used in a morally significant way without her consent. If Peter is wronged in becoming a parent against his will, so too a woman is wronged if forced to become a parent against her will.

A woman is certainly wronged if an agent impregnates her against her will, say through rape or through the implantation of an embryo in her uterus. It is important to remember that the rapist who impregnates her wrongs her. By contrast, the human being in utero is not an agent who is voluntarily making use of his or her mother's body against her will. Likewise, an infant can cause *harm* to someone (say, by disrupting a person's sleep), but an infant cannot *wrong* anyone (since to wrong someone requires deliberate action).

How then do we deal with allotting the responsibilities of parenthood in the scenarios envisioned by Smajdor and Cutas? One way out of the thicket is to put the ethical responsibility of "parenthood" on those who knowingly and willingly created the new human beings, namely the laboratory technicians and those who brought the laboratory technicians the genetic material. They are the ones who generate new human life, so they bear responsibility for the human beings that they produce.

There is a serious problem with this proposal, namely that it could diffuse parenthood too widely. Part of the advantage of having two parents is that the responsibilities of parenthood are shared, since it is difficult if not impossible for one person to provide all that a child needs physically, financially, psychologically, and spiritually. But having just *two* parents focuses the responsibility. Ten, twenty, or even more lab technicians may create human beings through artificial gametes working with genetic material secured from ten, twenty, or even more people. Suppose a "reproductive team" of forty people worked to make a child. It is impractical that all forty can reasonably share joint responsibility for the child. Just as a public park owned by everyone tends to receive less detailed attention than a private garden, so too would a child whose parents are the reproductive team likely to be no one's child. What belongs to everyone belongs to no one in particular, and children need particular people deeply invested in their well-being.

The scenario of more than two people becoming genetic parents to one child is explicitly envisioned and endorsed by César Palacios-González, John Harris, and Giuseppe Testa in their article "Multiplex Parenting: IVG and the Generations to Come." It is theoretically possible, making use of human embryonic stem cell (hESC) lines, that more than two people could become parents in a genetic sense to a single child. They explain: "Imagine that four people in a relationship want to parent a child while being all genetically related to her. IVG would enable the following scenario: first, two embryos would be generated from either couple through IVF with either naturally or in vitro generated gametes. hESC lines would be then established from both embryos and differentiated into IVG to be used in a second round of IVF. The resulting embryo would be genetically related to all four prospective parents, who would technically be the child's genetic grandparents."[11]

The same technology that would enable four people to become genetic parents to a child could also enable fourteen, forty, or four hundred to become genetic "parents" (or technically genetic great-grandparents) to a single child. Why would a group of people want to do such a thing? Well, I imagine most people would not want to do such a thing, but in the big world there are almost always groups of people who want to do what has never been done. Palacios-González, Harris, and Testa note, "If we find it morally unproblematic that people who cannot achieve natural reproduction rely on assisted reproduction to have genetically related kin then we find no reason why this should not hold also for non-couple partnerships for whom simultaneous genetic kinship is currently prevented, given that they will provide the necessary parenting and care for the resulting children."[12] We should deny the antecedent rather than embrace the absurd.

Another "bonus," on the view advocated by Palacios-González, Harris, and Testa, is that artificial gametes would facilitate consumer choice of a variety of potential children. It is easy to imagine such a future.

"Would you like your child between 6'1" and 6'2"?" asks the smiling salesperson. She continues with a friendly lilt in her voice, "We have a blond, blue-eyed one available with a 135 IQ. He has athletic potential for varsity high school basketball. Would this work for you, sir?"

"Well, I'm not sure. Let me run this by the others," sighs the reproductive committee chairperson. He texts a brief message on his phone before continuing, "Some of my potential co-parents were hoping for a little more intelligence, even if we have to downgrade the athletic ability. How much would it be to create a few hundred more embryos and try again?"

She frowns.

He exhales, then says, "I might have enough votes to make this option work for us. But I'll have to sell it to some members of the parental co-op. How good-looking will this product, I mean, child be? We don't have to have supermodel looks, which I know cost extra, but we need at least B-list model attractiveness."

This brave new world, even if populated with only beautiful people, is an ugly creation in which the gift of a child becomes a consumer product for committee consumption.

Four

Is *Roe v. Wade* Unquestionably Correct?

FEW, IF ANY, UNITED STATES SUPREME COURT DECISIONS HAVE GENERATED more controversy than its 1973 decision *Roe v. Wade*. In the *Washington Post* "Fact Checker" section, Michelle Ye Hee Lee reported on her investigation of the question, "Is the United States one of seven countries that 'allow elective abortions after 20 weeks of pregnancy'?" She found that "this statistic seemed dubious at first, because it seemed extreme for just seven countries out of 198 to allow elective abortions after 20 weeks of pregnancy. But upon further digging, the data back up the claim."[1] The law of the United States on abortion, grounded in *Roe*, is more extreme than almost every nation on earth.

UC Berkeley law dean Erwin Chemerinsky and Michele Goodwin make a case in their fifty-nine-page article "Abortion: A Woman's Private Choice" that US abortion law is not radical enough.[2] They hold that legalized abortion in the United States is in "serious jeopardy" and that we need to act now not only to preserve the law as it stands but to expand abortion rights. Chemerinsky and Goodwin write, "So-called 'informed consent' laws, special waiting periods for abortions, and prohibitions of 'partial birth abortions' all should be deemed unconstitutional."[3] More-over, the government should fund abortions, since failure to pay for abortion is "coercing motherhood upon poor, pregnant women."[4] They hold that the Supreme Court's most controversial case of all time is "un-questionably correct."[5] How do they justify this view?

Should the state forbid abortion or let women decide whether to abort? According to Chemerinsky and Goodwin, there is no consensus about when human life begins, nor does science clarify the matter:

> Why leave the choice as to abortion to the woman rather than to the state? First, there was then, and is now, no consensus as to when human life begins. As Professor Tribe explains: "The reality is that the 'general agreement' posited . . . simply does not exist." In other words, "Some regard the fetus as merely another part of the woman's body until quite late in pregnancy or even until birth; others believe the fetus must be regarded as a helpless human child from the time of its conception." Moreover, according to Professor Tribe, "These differ-ences of view are endemic to the historical situation in which the abortion controversy arose." The choice of conception as the point at which human life begins, which underlies state laws prohibiting abor-tion, thus was based not on consensus or science, but religious views.[6]

In their article, Chemerinsky and Goodwin show no awareness of the relevant scientific research about the beginning of an individual human being's life. Patrick Lee and Melissa Moschella summarize the relevant scientific findings:

> The following are typical examples—only three of the many, many we could cite. These are from standard texts by embryologists, devel-opmental biologists, and microbiologists:
> "Human life begins at fertilization, the process during which a male gamete or sperm unites with a female gamete or oocyte (ovum) to form a single cell called a zygote. This highly specialized, totipotent cell marked the beginning of each of us as a unique individual." "A zygote is the beginning of a new human being (i.e., an embryo)." Keith L. Moore, *The Developing Human: Clinically Oriented Embry-ology*, 7th edition.

"Fertilization is the process by which male and female haploid gametes (sperm and egg) unite to produce a genetically distinct individual." Signorelli et al., Kinases, phosphatases and proteases during sperm capacitation, *Cell Tissue Research*.

"Although life is a continuous process, fertilization (which, incidentally, is not a 'moment') is a critical landmark because, under ordinary circumstances, *a new, genetically distinct human organism is formed* when the chromosomes of the male and female pronuclei blend in the oocyte" (emphasis added; Ronan O'Rahilly and Fabiola Mueller, *Human Embryology and Teratology*, 3rd edition). Many other examples could be cited.[7]

The recognition that an individual human life begins at conception is a matter of science, not religious views or political ideology.

In another example, Sarah Knapton, the science editor of the *Telegraph*, notes, "Human embryos have been kept alive in a petri dish for an unprecedented 13 days, allowing scientists to finally see what happens in the mysterious days after implantation in the womb."[8] Only if human embryos are *already alive* can human embryos be *kept alive* for longer than ever before. Honest and informed defenders of abortion often concede that an individual living human being comes into existence at completed fertilization. For example, Kate Greasley writes, "All embryos and fetuses are certainly human beings, in that they are all individual human organisms."[9] By contrast, Chemerinsky and Goodwin exhibit science denial. It is not a sign of intellectual rigor to simply ignore scientific evidence.

Nor is it a sign of intellectual rigor to distort your opponents' positions. Chemerinsky and Goodwin write, "Legislatures could cloak religious objections to abortion in secular arguments (and often they do this) by claiming that potential human life exists at the point of conception."[10] They cite no scholar who holds this position. In fact, I am aware of no contemporary prolife advocate who claims that abortion is wrong because it kills *potential* human life. Rather, contemporary critics of abortion hold that abortion kills an actual human being with potential.

Chemerinsky and Goodwin's misrepresentation of prolife argumentation continues, "According to this line of argument, absent an abortion, all or the overwhelming majority of pregnancies develop fetuses to term and produce babies. This is woefully misguided and inaccurate."[11] After extensive reading of the literature on abortion, I know of no one who holds this position. Chemerinsky and Goodwin go on to critique this straw man by noting:

> Roughly 10%–20% of known pregnancies will spontaneously terminate, resulting in miscarriages. Moreover, two-thirds "of all human embryos fail to develop successfully," and terminate before women even know they are pregnant. Even in the most controlled, hormone-rich circumstances, such as in vitro fertilization—over 65% of the embryos end in demise. According to the most recent Centers For Disease Control and Prevention (CDC) data on this issue, only 23.5% of implanted embryos result in normal live births (for women over thirty-five years old, the chances of pregnancy resulting in live birth are dramatically lower). In other words, there is not a probable chance that but for an abortion there will be a baby resulting from conception. Instead, there may be a reasonable chance—but clearly no more than that—that there will be a baby but for an abortion.[12]

This is a red herring argument. Embryos that spontaneously abort before women even know they are pregnant are completely irrelevant for the abortion debate, since abortion cannot be chosen until pregnancy is known. Likewise, the fact that only 23.5 percent of implanted IVF embryos result in normal live births is irrelevant for the abortion debate. Women who go to the trouble and expense of implanting IVF embryos are women who want to be pregnant. Might some of these women change their minds midpregnancy? Perhaps, but such abortions are possible only if the embryos do not spontaneously miscarry. If Chemerinsky and Goodwin are correct that 10 to 20 percent of known pregnancies spontaneously terminate, that means 80 to 90 percent of known pregnancies continue to live birth. In other words, there is an excellent chance that a known pregnancy will result in a newborn unless an abortion takes place.

Chemerinsky and Goodwin's argument from spontaneous miscarriage is a red herring argument for another reason. The probability of survival of an individual is irrelevant to the question of whether that individual has the right to live. In some times and places, a majority of newborns died. In some times and places, a majority of AIDS victims did not survive. The probability of an individual's survival is irrelevant to the question of whether an individual has basic human rights.

Chemerinsky and Goodwin go on to point out that arguments against abortion based on "potential life" could just as well apply to contraception, which also acts against potential life. They write, "Arguments framed in protecting 'potential life' to justify a ban on contraceptives make as little sense [*sic*] they do when applied to abortion. However, the Catholic Church takes this position."[13]

It is true that some Catholic authors, such as Germain Grisez, argue that contraception is wrong because it is contralife.[14] But Grisez recognized that contraception and abortion differ morally in that abortion ends an actual human life while contraception prevents a human life from beginning.[15] In fact, the Catholic Church argues that abortion is wrong because it kills an (actual) human being, not "potential life." As the *Catechism of the Catholic Church* notes, not potential but actual "human life must be respected and protected absolutely from the moment of conception. From the first moment of his existence, a human being must be recognized as having the rights of a person—among which is the inviolable right of every innocent being to life."[16] The Catholic Church does indeed oppose contraception, but not because it prevents "potential life," a term that does not appear in the *Catechism*. Rather, "This particular doctrine, expounded on numerous occasions by the Magisterium, is based on the inseparable connection, established by God, which man on his own initiative may not break, between the unitive significance and the procreative significance which are both inherent to the marriage act."[17] Though the Catholic Church condones neither abortion nor contraception, the Church does not hold that they are wrong for the same reason.

After their examination of a straw-man version of one prolife argument, Chemerinsky and Goodwin conclude, "When examined closely, as we have here, Professor Tribe's argument that there is no secular basis for a prohibition on abortion and contraception makes profound sense."[18] It is not simply that Chemerinsky and Goodwin misunderstand the prolife view as articulated in the scholarly literature. Entirely missing from their analysis is any engagement with—indeed they show no awareness of—the many secular (nonreligious, nontheological) arguments advanced against abortion by scholars such as (atheist) Don Marquis, Robert P. George,

Patrick Lee, Francis Beckwith, and a host of others over the last decades.[19] In ignoring such authors, Chemerinsky and Goodwin provide an ostrich defense of abortion. It is easy to think *Roe*'s legalization of abortion is "unquestionably correct" when one simply ignores the questions raised by critics.

Not all defenders of abortion ignore prolife critics. In his article "A Present Like Ours," Michael Davis's challenges are not only to Don Marquis's future-like-ours critique of abortion but also to abortion critiques from the (new and classic) natural law perspective based on the person as an individual substance of a rational nature.[20] Davis writes, "Marquis's theory treats the rights of adult women as counting no more than those of a fetus no more complicated than an ameba. Even many people who oppose abortion will recognize that as discriminating against women."[21]

In fact, the prolife view does not treat the rights of adult women as counting no more than those of a fetus no more complicated than an amoeba. Women (and men) have numerous rights, both legally and morally, that are not enjoyed by a prenatal human being. They can drive, vote, run for public office, and, within the parameters of the law and sound ethics, govern their own lives in ways that no minor child may. The prolife view is not that women and unborn human beings have equal rights in every respect but that all human beings, born and unborn, male and female, mature and immature, share in the same basic rights, including the right to life. To treat all human beings as fundamentally equal in basic dignity is to avoid unjust discrimination by acknowledging that all women, all children, and all men are created equal and endowed with basic rights. Indeed, it is discrimination to treat some human beings—those who are not like us in terms of race, religion, or birth—as lacking basic rights. So it is not defenders of prenatal human beings but defenders of abortion who are acting to reinforce discrimination.

But the claim that all human beings have equal rights itself causes other problems on Davis's view:

> There are few, if any, places in the world today, or at any other time, where the criminal law would treat as a murderer the woman who deliberately obtained an early abortion. Even where abortion has been prohibited, the law has generally treated the fetus, even a relatively

mature fetus, as something less than "one of us." Marquis's theory proves more than it should. Marquis owes us an explanation of why abortion, even early in pregnancy, is not simple murder, deserving death or at least long imprisonment; or, if Marquis actually thinks it is murder, he should say so openly, accepting that as a conclusion against common sense.[22]

What he is saying is that if prolife advocates really believe that a prenatal human being has a right to life, then they should advocate for laws that make abortion not just a crime but a crime equal to first-degree murder.

If all human beings share in equal basic rights, does it follow that abortion must be treated by criminal law as first-degree murder? Should women who get abortions get the death penalty, be imprisoned for life, or at least be subjected to the same punishment as other people who intentionally kill innocent human beings? Are Marquis, and other defenders of the equal rights of prenatal human beings, fundamentally inconsistent in not making this demand? Or are prolife people lacking in forthrightness because they think women who get abortions should be treated as murderers but lack the courage to state this publicly?

Inconsistency and timidity are not the only alternatives. To defend the basic equal rights of all human beings does not necessarily mean that abortion should be punished as first-degree murder. Abortion and the murder of an adult are alike in that both involve the intentional killing of an innocent person. But there are also many important differences between an abortion and a typical case of murder. The first difference has to do with culpability in terms of knowledge and in terms of voluntariness. If I kill my auto mechanic, it is implausible in the extreme for me to try to excuse my act by claiming that I did not realize that he was an innocent human being. By contrast, in many (maybe even most) cases of abortion, the woman obtaining the abortion does not believe that her choice is terminating the life of an innocent human being. This ignorance could be culpable or inculpable, but ignorance of the personhood identity of the victim is almost never involved in typical cases of murder.

Second, the voluntariness of the act is often mitigated by great fear or anxiety on the part of the woman. When mothers kill their own newborns, as sometimes happens, it is not unusual for the punishment due for killing an innocent person to be mitigated in light of subjective factors that led to the killing, such as postpartum depression. Of course, abortion occurs antepartum, but by similar reasoning, mothers who authorize an abortion are often motivated by subjective factors such as intense fear, which reduces the voluntariness of the act. In many cases of abortion, again unlike typical cases of murder, duress is involved, in which the father of the child, and sometimes others, pressure the woman into getting an abortion that she would have never gotten had the news of the pregnancy been greeted with joy.

Third, the victim of abortion—although fundamentally equal—is not equal in all respects to the victim in a typical murder. In a typical murder, the victim's death negatively affects the victim's relatives and friends. The victim can no longer carry out his or her responsibilities at work or at home. The killing involved in murder may also make other people fear for their lives. The typical murder also brings a loss for all those who contributed to the life of the one who is killed—such as the parents, caregivers, and teachers who helped the victim gain maturity. Finally, the typical murder thwarts the life plans of the victim, whose dreams, ambitions, and plans are demolished by death.

These characteristics, typical of a case of murder, are not present in an abortion. A prenatal human being does not have friends, and relatives may not even know of his or her existence. Human beings who find out about someone else's abortion do not fear for their own lives, since abortions kill only prenatal human beings. An unborn child does not have responsibilities at work or home on which others depend. Only one person—the pregnant woman—has contributed to the maturation of the fetus, and this is the person who is authorizing the abortion. Moreover, the prenatal human being does not yet have plans, ambitions, and dreams that are thwarted by getting killed. So although the killing involved in abortion and the killing involved in a typical murder are the same in the most important fundamental sense—an innocent person's life is extinguished—in many other ways they are not the same. It makes sense, therefore, for the law to take these many differences into account when determining the punishment appropriate for abortion and appropriate for typical murder. These differences also answer the question of why it makes sense to rescue one five-year-old girl rather than ten frozen human embryos.

By similar reasoning, the assassination of the president of the United States should be treated more severely by law than the murder of a regular citizen, in virtue of the president's role in society and that fact that the president's death adversely affects not just immediate family members and friends but potentially the entire world. So, too, the murder of a regular person should be treated more severely by law than the intentional killing of a human being prior to birth. Yet making such differentiations is consistent with holding that in terms of basic human dignity the president, the regular citizen, and the human fetus have equal basic rights. It is not inconsistent for a defender of prenatal human beings to advocate lesser penalties for abortion than for the murder of postnatal human beings.

Moreover, prudential considerations of the enforceability of the law suggest that the penalties for violating laws forbidding abortion should fall on abortionists rather than on women getting abortions. Mitigating factors typically reduce the culpability of women seeking abortions. Abortionists ending the lives of prenatal human beings typically perform their tasks as part of a regular routine, without mitigating factors. If women were also subject to criminal penalties, it would make the prosecution of abortions much more difficult, since women would be implicating themselves in criminal activity by testifying against the abortionists. Moreover, abortionists typically kill many prenatal human beings, whereas an individual woman rarely has many abortions. With laws against illegal drugs, the law should focus on the drug dealers who profit from endangering others rather than on the drug users who often suffer from their use. Similarly, laws against abortion should focus on abortionists who profit from killing rather than on women who often suffer from abortions.

In another critique of the prolife view, Robert Lovering's "The Substance View: A Critique (Part 2)" casts the prolife view as resting on "the basic potential for rational moral agency" of the prenatal human being.[23] But the prolife view in its standard articulations by Robert George, Francis Beckwith, Patrick Lee, and many others, including myself, rests on the claim, not that every human being prior to birth has the basic potential for rational moral agency, but rather that every human being (born and unborn) actually (not just potentially) possesses a rational nature.[24] What is the difference? A basic potential for rational agency may not be present in some human beings, such as those who have a serious mental handicap.

Yet such human beings deserve fundamental protection against exploitation and against being intentionally killed.

Having misrepresented the prolife position, Lovering points out that "it's very difficult to see how this unactualizable potential could confer moral standing. For all practical purposes, there is no difference between possessing this unactualizable potential and not possessing it at all. Given this, it's very difficult to see how there could be a *moral* difference between possessing this unactualizable potential and not possessing it at all."[25] The difficulty arises only because the rational nature of a being is confused with its actual potential for rational agency.

But perhaps this response only pushes the dispute to a different level. Why should we say that a particular being has a rational nature if in fact this being has no actual potential to perform rational activities? This question might be clarified in the course of considering another objection to the substance view.

Lovering notes that if we hold that human beings prior to birth have a basic potential for rational moral agency because most or many of them will develop to the point where they possess either proximate or immediately exercisable rational agency, then a problem arises. Because an estimated 60 percent of pregnancies end in spontaneous miscarriage, only 40 percent of prenatal human beings will ever exercise rational agency. If we hold that 40 percent or even a much lower percentage of successful development of rational agency is sufficient, then we are acting arbitrarily and moving closer to the view that rational agency is irrelevant.[26]

Even assuming that 60 percent of pregnancies spontaneously miscarry, this argument is problematic. To examine this objection, let's consider what it is to be a mammal. Part of what distinguishes mammals is the ability to nurse their young. So human beings, dogs, and zebras are mammals; iguanas, tapeworms, and wasps are not mammals. Not so fast, replies the critic. Do you not realize that some human beings, dogs, and zebras do not nurse their young, even cannot nurse their young? Male mammals of all these species cannot nurse their young, females before puberty cannot nurse their young, and elderly females cannot nurse their young. There are even cases of females of reproductive age who cannot nurse their young. The percentage of human beings, dogs, and zebras capable of nursing their young is, therefore, well below 40 percent. So are we mistaken in claiming that all human beings are mammals?

Of course not. In fact, all human beings, dogs, and zebras are mammals, not just females of those species and not just females of reproductive age, because all these creatures belongs to the kind of species that nurses its young. So, too, there is nothing arbitrary about including prenatal human beings in the category of rational animals.

In his *Scholastic Metaphysics* (required reading for anyone interested in the intersection of classic Thomistic metaphysics and analytic philosophy), Edward Feser clarifies what is at issue: "The distinction between essence and properties makes sense of the distinction between normal and defective instances. . . . Given its essence, a cat has four legs, but this property might not manifest itself in a particular cat if the cat is genetically or otherwise damaged. . . . Its lack of four legs just makes it a defective cat, and precisely because four-leggedness is one of its properties."[27] Feser goes on to point out that all human beings are rational animals, even if some human beings, because of genetic malfunction, brain injury, or immaturity, do not engage in rational activity. Indeed, we identify this human being as immature, or brain damaged, or genetically malformed because we have already properly categorized him or her as a rational animal. The defect points to the nondefective; immaturity is understood by reference to maturity.

Now consider another objection to the substance view offered by Lovering. Imagine that scientists discover a rational agency serum that can boost the intelligence of chimpanzees so they are like the apes in *Planet of the Apes*. These chimps would clearly be persons with rights to live. "Now, clearly, the ultimate potential for rational moral agency in their case would be an accidental property," writes Lovering, who concludes, "It's not the case, then, that an entity's moral standing *must* be a function of its essential properties."[28] An entity's moral standing, as in the case of these apes, can rest on accidental properties.

This objection rests on the assertion that the apes in the sci-fi example have acquired their standing as rational agents because of an accidental quality. I disagree. That some apes were injected with the rationality serum may be accidental in some senses. For example, maybe, much like penicillin, the rational agency serum was found by accident rather than by a deliberate plan to create rational agents. The property in question could also be accidental in that these apes rather than other apes were injected. Perhaps the scientists injected whichever apes happened to be on one side of the cage, or perhaps they injected a particular ape if a flipped quarter landed heads but not if it landed tails. The apes may have an accidental property in these senses, but in another sense (the sense presumably meant by Lovering) the property in question cannot be accidental. The rationality serum causes not an accidental but rather a substantial change in the ape. The ape, in virtue of gaining radically new abilities, becomes a radically different kind of creature with a radically different moral status. Just as an injection that kills an ape brings about substantial change in the ape from living to deceased, so too (if such a thing is even possible) the rational agency serum would bring about a substantial change transforming the individual from an ape to something radically new.

Lovering also raises a dilemma against the substance view. Do dolphins, apes, and whales have intrinsic value or extrinsic value? He writes, "By 'intrinsic' value I mean value it's logically possible for something to have even if it were the only thing that existed."[29] If there were only one person, that person would have intrinsic value. But if there were only one toothbrush, that toothbrush would not have intrinsic value, and it would gain extrinsic value only if there were people who liked to have clean teeth. Moreover, we can say that intrinsic value does not come in degree: a being either has it or does not have it. Extrinsic value, again by contrast, may come in degrees (the toothbrush is more or less useful, more or less valuable depending upon the circumstances). If intrinsic value does not come in degrees, then dolphins, apes, whales and other intelligent animals either have moral status just like us (which advocates of the substance view reject) or have no intrinsic value at all (which is counterintuitive, "given their similarities to beings with the ultimate potential for rational moral agency").[30] On the other hand, if such creatures are to have only extrinsic value, then they have the same moral status as tools, which also seems counterintuitive because almost everyone condemns animal cruelty.

If nonrational animals do not have equal moral status with human beings, does it follow that they are mere tools with which human agents can do anything they please? This conclusion does not follow. Let's say that someone legally obtained Michelangelo's *Pietà* and decided to destroy it for no good reason. Would this action be ethically problematic? Yes, you might maintain, because it would deprive innumerable people of the chance to see this beautiful sculpture. So let's say the owner of the *Pietà* was the last man in the world: could he destroy it then for no good reason? The *Pietà* is, after all, a mere piece of marble and so lacks intrinsic value. True, but the man who destroyed it would be acting badly inasmuch as it is against reason to destroy something of spectacular beauty without sufficient reason. A reasonable response to a thing of beauty is to contemplate and cherish it, not destroy it. If Aquinas is right, acting against reason is ethically wrong.[31]

On the other hand, if the man had to break apart the *Pietà* to make a barricade so that wild animals wouldn't eat him, he would be justified in destroying the statue. In a similar way, a reasonable response to potential or actual suffering is to alleviate it. Just as beauty is something in general to be contemplated and cherished, suffering is something in general to be avoided and minimized. It is unreasonable to inflict pain on a sentient being without sufficient justification. To delight in inflicting pain is irrational. So unless a person has a sufficient justification for inflicting pain on an animal, an agent is unjustified in doing so. Animal cruelty is therefore wrong, but we don't need to assume that animals have rights (any more than statues have rights) in order to come to this judgment.[32]

Unlike defenders of abortion such as Lovering who examine actual prolife arguments, Chemerinsky and Goodwin do not show awareness of the relevant literature. Perhaps for this reason, they also seem to regard the fetus as merely another part of the woman's body.[33] They confuse being *inside* someone's body with being a *part* of someone's body. An in vitro embryo is inside the glass petri dish but is not a part of the glass petri dish. Similarly, the prenatal human being is inside the woman's body but is not a part of her body. The prenatal human being often has a different blood type, race, and sex than the woman. Are we supposed to believe that the body of a pregnant woman has four legs, two heads, and half the time a penis? If the human being in utero is simply a part of the woman's body, how can we account for cases, such as some car accidents, in which she dies but her child survives? Save in cases of transplantation, parts of my body do not survive my death.

Moreover, even if the prenatal human being were just part of the woman's body, the right of a person to decide what happens to her body is limited in innumerable ways. We cannot appear naked in public, use meth, have sex in the street, or sell ourselves into slavery. Our moral and legal rights to use our bodies are limited also by the bodies of other people. There is no right to use one's body in such a way that it harms another human being's body. Chemerinsky and Goodwin cite the Tuskegee study of untreated syphilis as shameful experiments on vulnerable human populations. They are right. But Chemerinsky and Goodwin are not consistent advocates for vulnerable human populations, since they wish to exclude human beings in utero from legal protection.

Chemerinsky and Goodwin point out that the state cannot compel a person to use her body to keep another person alive.[34] It is illegal to force someone to donate blood or bone marrow, even if the blood or bone marrow is necessary to keep another person, even one's own son or daughter, alive. "Just as the law does not require individuals to donate body organs to save other people's lives, so should the state not require a woman to donate her body, against her will, to house a fetus."[35] So, they argue, the state cannot force a woman to keep the human being in utero alive by forbidding abortion.

The principle at issue—forcing one person to use his or her body in order to help another person—does not support abortion, unless one assumes that the fetal person is a nonentity. If the prenatal human being has human rights, then the principle of not using the body of one individual to help another is a principle that supports a prolife position. If it is wrong to force one human being to give up some of her blood in order to save the life of another human being, then it is even more problematic to force one human being (the one in utero) to give up all of her blood, all her organs, and her life itself, not to save the life of another person, but to render another person free of pregnancy. In the case of abortion, what the donor gives up is much more substantial (life itself) and what the recipient receives is much less substantial than life itself (freedom from pregnancy). So if forced organ donation is wrong to save someone's life, then it is even more problematic to end someone's life to free someone from pregnancy.

Chemerinsky and Goodwin, moreover, show little evidence of familiarity with the relevant literature in terms of defenses of abortion. They write, "Although everyone can agree that an individual capable of surviving outside the womb should be protected, consensus never will be reached as to the status of the fetus."[36] Many defenders of abortion disagree. Michael Tooley, Peter Singer, Alberto Giubilini, and Francesca Minerva disagree that an individual capable of surviving outside the womb should be protected. They have defended abortion and infanticide on the grounds that both the newborn and the prenatal human being are not "persons" in the ethically relevant sense.[37]

Indeed, the many defenses of infanticide over the last forty years suggest that consensus may never be reached about the status of the newborn.[38] If we adopt the principle endorsed by Chemerinsky and Goodwin that lack of consensus grounds the liberty to choose termination of young human life, then we should endorse both abortion and infanticide. If, on the other hand, the lack of consensus about newborn personhood is irrelevant for protecting in law and respecting the life of every infant, then lack of consensus would also seem irrelevant for fetal personhood.

An argument repeated in "Abortion: A Women's Private Choice" is that criminalization of abortion is especially burdensome for poor women and that a disproportionate number of the poor are minorities. If abortion is made illegal, rich white women will still be able to obtain abortions by going abroad.[39]

Indeed, the rich have an easier time evading all laws than do the poor. If O. J. Simpson had been an economically disadvantaged, unknown person, he would probably have been convicted of murder. Rich people can fly to other countries for the sake of evading US law against child prostitution, but it hardly follows from this fact that we should decriminalize child prostitution. Rich white women are less likely to get traffic tickets than poor black women, but we should not therefore abolish traffic laws. Legal justice should be blind to race and to class, but this is a problem for those responsible for enforcement of the legal system in general and, therefore, irrelevant for laws about abortion specifically.

In sum, Chemerinsky and Goodwin's defense of legal abortion does not take into account, let alone engage and refute, scholarly arguments from a prolife perspective. They highlight the risks that women will encounter if abortion is criminalized and ignore the harms that abortion causes women. They repeat the claim that abortion is more dangerous than childbirth and ignore evidence to the contrary.[40] Chemerinsky and Goodwin's article on abortion attacks straw men, employs red herrings, and ignores relevant evidence. "Abortion: A Woman's Private Choice" is very much in the spirit of *Roe*.

Five

What Are Reproductive Rights?

IN COMMON PARLANCE, SYNONYMS FOR *REPRODUCTIVE RIGHTS* INCLUDE *reproductive autonomy, reproductive justice,* or, even more euphemistically, *women's health.* But what exactly are reproductive rights? What are the scope and limits (if any) of reproductive rights? What is the basis for the legal and moral duties that come with reproducing? This chapter examines reproductive rights.

RIVAL DEFINITIONS OF REPRODUCTIVE RIGHTS

A fruitful conversation about such questions can begin with a disambiguation of the term *reproductive rights.* Part of the ambiguity hinges on the adjective *reproductive.* What is the object of reproductive rights? That is, what is the precise claim that advocates of reproductive rights assert? The proposed objects of reproductive rights include but are not limited to the following: access to abortion, contraception, and reproductive technologies such as IVF and cloning, as well as the freedom to perform sexual acts of a reproductive kind. Some understand reproductive rights to be the freedom to have genetically related offspring; others consider it the freedom to rear one's genetic offspring.[1]

Many authors distinguish the liberty to reproduce and the liberty not to reproduce.[2]

As used in political debates, the term *reproductive rights* is a common euphemism for the ability to access abortion and contraception, the liberty not to reproduce. But this liberty is no longer possible when someone is in the pursuit of an abortion. At least if the arguments of the last chapter are correct, abortion involves the termination of the life of a living human being: that is, abortion involves destroying the fruit of completed reproduction. Once a woman is pregnant, reproduction has been accomplished. Abstinence from sexual intercourse, the use of contraception, and not treating infertility can rightly be understood as actions that are not reproductive, but abortion cannot. In any case, the following reflections focus on the liberty not to reproduce rather than the liberty to reproduce.

Another part of the ambiguity in speaking about reproductive rights arises from the multiple meanings of the term *rights*. Making use of the work of Wesley Hohfeld, John Finnis distinguishes a liberty right from a claim right.[3] A liberty right (also called a privilege right) to X is the proposition that the person in question has no duty not to X. For example, if a person has a right to travel to Tulsa, this means that the person has no legal or ethical duty to refrain from going to Tulsa. In contrast, if an agent has a claim right, then other agents have a duty to either positively aid or negatively refrain from interfering with a person's having or doing X. An agent's right to live is a negative claim right, which means that other people have the duty not to intentionally kill the agent. A child's right to due care, a positive claim right, means that other people, namely the parents, have a duty to provide the necessities for the child's well-being. Some authors consider reproductive rights to be liberty rights; others consider them to be claim rights.[4]

Reproductive rights clearly cannot be the claim right of an individual person because reproduction (at least given current technology) involves the gametes of two people, so a single person cannot reproduce without the aid of another person (either in the act of sexual intercourse or through gamete donation). But everyone agrees that no one is morally or legally obligated to become a parent through either forcible intercourse or forcible donation of gametes. Presumably, this negative right of nonreproduction overrides any possible positive claim right of others to help us reproduce. In other words, if some person wanted to reproduce by means of sexual intercourse but could not find a willing partner, then that person wanting to reproduce through sexual intercourse would not have a positive claim right to reproduce.

A final cause of ambiguity is whether the term *reproductive rights* refers to legal rights or moral rights. In the United States, we have the legal right to be rude, uncaring, and cruel in speech to whomever we like, but we have no moral right to such conduct because we have a moral duty to refrain from hateful speech. Similarly, no one should be legally prevented by the force of law from having a child through governmental imposition of involuntary abortion or sterilization. However, there is no inconsistency in also insisting that no person has a moral right to have a child, or even to perform acts from which a child may arise. The disambiguation of the term *reproductive rights* is merely a first step in the debate, but it is a necessary first step for any meaningful discussion of the key questions arising from an assertion of a right to reproduce.

REPRODUCTIVE RIGHTS AND REPRODUCTIVE DUTIES

Much is written about reproductive rights, but comparatively little is written about reproductive duties. Yet important conceptual links characteristically exist between rights and corresponding duties. Muireann Quigley, in "A Right to Reproduce?," considers two justifications for reproductive rights: first, that they arise from an agent's interest in reproducing, and second, that they arise from autonomy.[5] She suggests that both justifications face serious difficulties. Part of the problem in considering reproductive rights in individualistic terms, somewhat articulated by Quigley, is that procreation is inherently other-regarding in two ways. First, at least given current technology, it always involves the gametes of two adults. Second, even if technology at some point in the future allowed one person to reproduce alone through cloning or the creation of gametes so that women could make sperm or men could make eggs, procreation would still be inherently social because procreation by definition brings about the life of someone else, another human person. When looking for justifications and limits to reproductive rights, the inherently social dimension of such liberty is often overlooked. To be a parent always involves a child. Quigley notes that Bonnie Steinbock thinks that the right to reproduce is not unrestricted but rather is limited to those who have an interest and ability to raise a child. This is, it seems to me, an absolutely necessary restriction on reproductive liberty understood in a moral sense.

Reproductive rights have to do with becoming a parent, and becoming a parent is necessarily linked to having children and thus accepting the duties that arise from having children. In her article "Parental Obligation," Nellie Wieland examines rival accounts of what grounds paternal and maternal duties.[6] One option is that parenting is a chosen substantive life project, but some people clearly count as parents who either have not taken up or have chosen to discontinue parenting as a life project. A father who abandons his family does not cease to be a father. He becomes a bad father. I agree with Wieland that such persons still have obligations to their children, so the choice of parenting as a life project cannot ground parental obligations.

A second option defines parenting as mere biological relation. Wieland rejects this option, asserting that mere biological relationships have no moral content and that a "biologically grounded obligation would also fail to explain the obligations that we readily assume are waived in the case of adoption, sperm and egg donorship, and, possibly, in cases of rape. Although a 'bare' biologically grounded obligation would be sweeping in its reach—children would be broadly covered by their biological parents—it fails to demonstrate that there is moral content in biological relation."[7]

The claim that bare biology is irrelevant to moral content is not a self-evident truth. Perhaps lurking in the background is the "is/ought" fallacy or the fact/value distinction, but these justifications for the claim are themselves highly questionable.[8] That someone is my biological brother or sister, or mother or father, seems highly relevant to how I should treat them in a variety of situations. To treat such a person as a perfect stranger indicates a lack of sensitivity to the familial duties that—though not chosen—are nevertheless real. The precise scope and specifications of these duties are matters for investigation, but the idea that biological relationships are irrelevant for ethics is—on the face of it—rather absurd. Should we really tell Oedipus Rex that he shouldn't worry a bit about killing his father and marrying his mother since, after all, he has mere biological relationships to them?

As for adoption, the obligation to care for children is not waived but rather discharged in securing a family for the adopted child. Sperm donation and egg donation are ethically problematic for a variety of reasons, one being that they deprive the children of the proper relationship to their biological parents. If a child has already been brought into existence, adoption may be the best way to ensure his or her proper care. But to cause a child to come into existence, knowing beforehand that the child will not have a social relationship with his or her biological mother, biological father, or both, is to wrong that child.

Finally, in rape, I believe the mother (in the biological and gestational senses of the term) does have obligations not to kill or otherwise intentionally or recklessly harm her biological child. Everyone has such obligations. After birth, she may choose to discharge her obligations to the child through placing the child for adoption, or she may choose to become a social mother (that is the female parent who raises the child). The case for understanding the duties of parenthood as based in biology is not undermined by Weiland's considerations.

Weiland notes a third option for grounding parental duties: "Biological parents, *being causally responsible for the existence of their children*, presumably inherit a moral responsibility to care adequately for their dependent children or to see that they are cared for by others. Generally speaking, parents have basic substantive reasons to give priority to their children's interests, reasons tied almost inextricably to biological relation. These reasons are substantive not because the biological relation in itself gives rise to them but because parents have brought into the world children who need care."[9]

This justification fails on Wieland's view, because "the complexities of reproductive voluntariness, autonomy and control are enough to cast doubt on many, if not most, cases."[10] I am not convinced this conclusion is correct, in part because, as just stated, many moral obligations do not arise simply because of our own voluntary, autonomous choice to take on the moral obligation.

What does ground parental obligation? On Weiland's view, it is the unique ability of parents to help and harm their own children. She says, "My argument will be relatively simple: (i) parents are in the best position to optimize the well-being of their children; (ii) those same parents are in the best position to cause harm to their children by not attempting to optimize this well-being; and (iii) children are deserving of moral regard. Therefore, (iv) parents have an obligation to care for their children even when it is costly, involuntary and unrewarding."[11]

Strictly speaking, this argument is a non sequitur since a logical term in the conclusion ("an obligation to care for their children even when it is costly, involuntary and unrewarding") does not appear in the premises. However, the conclusion of the argument is an interesting thesis worth considering.

A question for Weiland's reasoning is who exactly the "parents" are and why. As Robert Sparrow points out, there are numerous senses of the term, including "social parents, gestational parents, genetic parents, commissioning parents, causal parents, 'cytoplasmic' parents, and mitochondrial parents."[12] In the future, some children, argues Sparrow, may actually have no genetic parents at all: "I want to suggest that if an ovum derived from one embryonic stem cell line were fertilized using sperm derived from another embryonic stem cell line and if the embryo that resulted was then implanted into a woman's womb, then any child that was born would have no genetic parents! The child would, of course, have a gestational mother and may have social parents (one of whom may be the gestational mother). However, there would be no individuals, living or dead, who would have the appropriate genetic relationship to the child to be described as its genetic parent."[13]

Why not say that the original embryos from whom the gametes were derived are the genetic parents? Sparrow writes,

> It is true that these embryos are the only organisms with a genome in the appropriate informational relationship to the genome of the child to stand in the relation of "genetic parent." However, while they might serve as placeholders in a family tree, embryos cannot play either of the roles, discussed above, that we require of genetic parents. Individuals cannot interpret their lives and experiences in the light of

"biographies" of embryos. Institutions cannot assign responsibility for the care of children to embryos or consult embryos about the fate of embryos created with their gametes. More fundamentally, it is internal to the concept of parenthood that parents are persons, living or dead, who stand in the appropriate (social, gestational, causal, genetic, etc.) relationship to the child. Thus, I would suggest that to have embryos as genetic "parents" is to have no genetic parents at all. Instead, the children born of such matings might be said to be "orphaned" at conception.[14]

This argument fails. It is true that individuals cannot interpret their lives and experiences in the light of biographies of embryos, but the biographies of anonymous sperm donors or of ova taken from aborted female fetuses are equally unknown. It is true that institutions cannot assign responsibility for the care of children to embryos or consult embryos about the fate of embryos created with their gametes, but this is equally true of children whose fathers died before their birth. Finally, even if it is internal to the concept of parenthood that parents are persons, living or dead, who stand in the appropriate (social, gestational, causal, genetic, etc.) relationship to the child, in his "Orphaned at Conception: The Uncanny Offspring of Embryos" Sparrow simply assumes without argument the deeply controversial claim that human embryos cannot be persons.

The duties of reproduction are also explored in Mianna Lotz's article "Rethinking Procreation: Why It Matters Why We Have Children," which imagines three cases of malevolent conception in which people create new people in ways that profoundly disadvantage them:

Reckless Paula. While Paula is trying to become pregnant, she learns that, if she conceives a child now, there is a risk that it may have [a certain] handicap. If she waits two months before conceiving a child, there would be no such risk. She decides not to wait. As a result her child, Paul, is handicapped albeit not to an extent that would make his life not worth living.
The secretly ambitious lab technician. A secretly ambitious lab technician is deliberating whether to introduce a certain solution into a dish that contains a single egg and a single sperm cell. The technician is

aware that the solution will cause the baby produced by this union of egg and sperm to be born with a serious congenital disorder. However, the important research that the technician is conducting is on the effect that the solution will have on the developing embryo. So, if the technician's hand is stayed by law, morality, or some other force he will simply discard the contents of the dish. Suppose then that he drops the solution into the dish and does not discard the contents of the dish. . . . The embryo is returned to the womb of its genetic mother to develop, and the baby is in fact born with the serious congenital disorder but nonetheless has a life well worth living.

The malicious scientist. A malicious scientist employs genetic screening and in vitro fertilization to produce the most diseased, handicapped individual he can possibly produce who will nevertheless have a life just barely worth living—just to enjoy watching the suffering.[15]

Cases of malevolent conception raise interesting philosophical questions. Derek Parfit's nonidentity thesis holds that if someone otherwise would not exist, then that person is not harmed (where *harmed* means made worse off), even in cases of malevolent conception, by being brought into existence. Since such children would not have been at all, they cannot be harmed and so also are not wronged, save if "their life is not worth living." Making the same point, Joyce Havstad quotes Raanan Gillon: "What is preferable for that child? To exist but to have those problems, or not to exist at all?"[16] No harm is done, since the child is not made worse off.

In an appeal to the collective interests of the community, Lotz proposes a way to show what is wrong with cases of malevolent conception despite the nonidentity thesis, "To manifest an indifference to introducing avoidable suffering into one's community, is to show a lack of respect for the community itself, even if it cannot be said to be a disrespect shown to a specific, not-yet-existing member of that community. It is a disrespect that offends the community by undermining its regard for itself, and its valuing of itself." However, this principle may not work to explain the (presumed) wrongness of creating a gravely disadvantaged child if creating this child serves the good of the community. Ursula Le Guin's short story "The Ones Who Walk Away from the Omelas" and Lois Lowry's *The*

Giver offer literary depictions of situations in which community well-being is served, rather than undermined, by the suffering of a single child. Presumably, to create a gravely disadvantaged child is still wrong even if this creation is done for the service of the community. This solution, like appeal to impersonal principles, also fails to focus our moral attention where it should be: on the disadvantaged child, not on the community.

Six

Is It Better Never to Have Been Born?

HAVING THOUGHT ABOUT THE ABORTION ISSUE FOR DECADES, I SELDOM read an entirely new perspective. But the article examined in this chapter was for me strikingly novel. Dan Thomas's article "Better Never to Have Been Born: Christian Ethics, Anti-abortion Politics, and the Pro-life Paradox" makes the case that there is an inconsistency in the beliefs of Christian critics of abortion.[1] Even if the arguments of previous chapter are correct, Thomas argues that consistent Christians cannot embrace an opposition to abortion.

Christian belief holds that all human beings have one of two ultimate destinies: heaven or hell. To go to hell is the worst possible fate for a human being; to go to heaven is the best possible fate. So what determines whether a human being goes to heaven or to hell? According to Thomas's account of Christian belief, "Damnation can only be conferred on moral agents who can act of their own accord and thus willingly accept or reject God's grace."[2] Now all human beings prior to the age of reason—for example, toddlers, babies, and prenatal human beings—are not responsible agents who can be held ethically accountable for their actions. They cannot perform human actions as morally good or evil but only acts of a human being that cannot be evaluated ethically, such as breathing or circulating blood. If these beliefs are correct, Thomas continues, "the only way to avoid hell entirely is to come into existence briefly—for a few seconds, a few minutes, or a few years—and then die because an early death comes with an eternal safeguard: innocent children maintain their innocence forever."[3] Indeed, Thomas points out that Christians hold that life in heaven is infinitely more important than life on earth as well as infinitely longer in duration: "According to the author of the book of James, human life does not last very long: 'What is your life? For you are a mist that appears for a little while and then vanishes' (James 4:14). A blip, a bubble, a mist, a dream, a tiny speck, a poof of wind, a candle-snuff: such analogies appear throughout Christian literature and denote the transience of human existence."[4] It is madness to prefer life on earth to eternal life in heaven.

Given their theological suppositions, Christian prolife activists hold incompatible beliefs. "In their attempts to lengthen earthly lives," writes Thomas, "conservative activists endanger infant souls. For the sake of life on Earth, they jeopardize the assurance of Life in heaven."[5] Since the death of the newborn baby or the prenatal human being secures eternal life for him or her, consistent Christians should not condemn but rather celebrate both abortion and infanticide, since "death alone guarantees the infant's salvation."[6] Likewise, consistent Christians should not criticize but commend abortionists as bringing more people to heaven than anyone else. "If the unborn are indeed spiritually blameless, then abortion practitioners are not monstrous murderers. They are instead the nation's most effective evangelists. Under their supervision, abortees reap the benefits of being born again without ever being born at all."[7] In Thomas's view, given Christian beliefs about heaven and hell, "The only safe child is a dead one."[8] What Dan Thomas calls the "Pro-life Paradox" is the alleged inconsistency in Christian beliefs about the afterlife and Christian defense of prenatal human beings.

How might a Christian critic of abortion respond to Thomas's argument that "it is better not to be born"? If this argument were true, the Pro-life Paradox would also justify killing many normal adults. On the supposition that baptism takes away all sin and makes someone fit for heaven, should we not murder an adult immediately after her baptism? Why not wait outside a confessional and shoot someone in the head after his sins have been forgiven? Killing in these cases would assure that the person did not go to hell by later falling into mortal sin and dying in this condition. So murders of this kind should be celebrated as saving someone from the dangers of going to hell. This consequence is absurd. In the same way, so is the Pro-life Paradox. But where exactly does the Pro-life Paradox go wrong?

One key supposition in Dan Thomas's Pro-life Paradox is the presumption that all humans who die before the age of reason certainly go to heaven. But many Christian theologians, indeed most Christian theologians over the centuries, reject the presumption that infants and prenatal human beings who die certainly go to heaven. Three views are most prominent in the theological tradition.

First, Augustine of Hippo taught that unbaptized infants go to hell, where they receive the lightest punishment possible because they have only original sin and no actual sin.[9] St. Jerome, St. Gregory the Great, and St. Anselm agreed. If these theologians are right, then abortionists not only kill the unborn but also consign them to hell. The only way infants can avoid hell is if they are born.

St. Thomas Aquinas proposed a second option in which infants dying without baptism enjoy a natural happiness, which he called "limbo," that differs from heavenly supernatural happiness.[10] St. Gregory of Nyssa, St. Bonaventure, and Bl. Duns Scotus held similar views. If these theologians are right, then abortionists not only deprive human beings in utero of earthly life but also ensure that they will not have heavenly life. Although the natural happiness of limbo is possible, the only way infants can go to heaven is if they are allowed to be born.

A third option is that we simply do not know with certainty what happens to children who die before the age of reason without baptism, but we can hope that somehow they are saved. The *Catechism of the Catholic Church* expresses this view:

> As regards *children who have died without Baptism*, the Church can only entrust them to the mercy of God, as she does in her funeral rites for them. Indeed, the great mercy of God who desires that all men

should be saved, and Jesus' tenderness toward children which caused him to say: "Let the children come to me, do not hinder them," allow us to hope that there is a way of salvation for children who have died without Baptism. All the more urgent is the Church's call not to prevent little children coming to Christ through the gift of holy Baptism.[11]

This view is also expressed by the Congregation for the Doctrine of the Faith in 1980 as well as the International Theological Commission in 2007.[12] It is important to note that the *Catechism of the Catholic Church* speaks of hope and that hope differs from presumption.[13] Hope concerns the good of salvation that is possible but difficult to obtain. By contrast, presumption assumes that salvation is a good that is not just possible to obtain but certain to happen. If the view expressed in the *Catechism of the Catholic Church* is correct, then it is presumption to assume with certainty that all unbaptized infants go to heaven, though we may hope that they do.

A fourth prominent view of who is saved also causes the prolife paradox to collapse. Avery Cardinal Dulles notes that "Clement of Alexandria, Origen, Gregory Nazianzen, and Gregory of Nyssa sometimes speak as though in the end all will be saved."[14] Dulles points out that in more recent times Edith Stein, Karl Rahner, Jacques Maritain, Richard John Neuhaus, and most famously Hans Urs von Balthasar defended the possibility that everyone escapes the pains of hell. If everyone escapes the pains of hell, then killing children before or after their birth deprives them of their lives on earth but is irrelevant to preventing their eternal damnation.

So if Augustine or Aquinas or the *Catechism of the Catholic Church* or Von Balthasar is correct about the fate of infants dying without baptism, then Dan Thomas's Pro-life Paradox collapses. But let's assume for the sake of argument that all four of these theological views are mistaken. Would Dan Thomas's case for the Pro-life Paradox then be justified?

The work of Thomas Aquinas can shed some light on this question. For Thomas, one must undergo baptism of water, blood, or desire in order to have eternal life.[15] In the *Summa theologiae*, Aquinas asks "whether children of Jews or other unbelievers should be baptized against the will of their parents."[16] His answer is that they should not be baptized (even though their eternal salvation is at stake) because it is contrary to natural justice to usurp the role of parents in governing their own children, in-

cluding determining whether their children are to be baptized. Nothing—
not even securing someone's salvation—justifies doing an unjust act.

In the very next article, Thomas asks "whether a child can be baptized
while yet in its mother's womb." Aquinas considers the objection, "Further, eternal death is a greater evil than death of the body. But of two evils
the less should be chosen. If, therefore, the child in the mother's womb
cannot be baptized, it would be better for the mother to be opened, and
the child to be taken out by force and baptized, than that the child should
be eternally damned through dying without Baptism."[17] In this objection,
Aquinas pithily summarizes the heart of Dan Thomas's Pro-life Paradox.

Aquinas critiques this objection by citing the Pauline Principle, "We
should 'not do evil that there may come good' (Rom. 3:8). Therefore it is
wrong to kill a mother that her child may be baptized. If, however, the
mother die while the child lives yet in her womb, she should be opened
that the child may be baptized."[18] The same reasoning applies to the case
of intentionally killing a child in utero in order to secure eternal life for
the child (though it is extremely hard to believe that abortions are actually
undertaken for the purpose of securing heavenly happiness for the child;
the motivation of the abortionist is not the child's eternal salvation but
money). The Pauline Principle that Aquinas articulates is absolutely fundamental: "It often happens that man acts with a good intention, but
without spiritual gain, because he lacks a good will. Let us say that someone robs in order to feed the poor: in this case, even though the intention
is good, the uprightness of the will is lacking. Consequently, no evil done
with a good intention can be excused. 'There are those who say: And why
not do evil that good may come? Their condemnation is just' (*Rom* 3:8)."[19]

Of course, an emphasis on the Pauline Principle not to do evil that
good may come is not something unique to the thought of Aquinas. In
Veritatis splendor, Pope St. John Paul II emphasized that the Pauline Principle is fundamental in the entire Christian tradition:

> In teaching the existence of intrinsically evil acts, the Church accepts
> the teaching of Sacred Scripture. The Apostle Paul emphatically states:
> "Do not be deceived: neither the immoral, nor idolaters, nor adulter-
> ers, nor sexual perverts, nor thieves, nor the greedy, nor drunkards,
> nor revilers, nor robbers will inherit the Kingdom of God" (1 *Cor*
> 6:9–10). If acts are intrinsically evil, a good intention or particular

circumstances can diminish their evil, but they cannot remove it. They remain "irremediably" evil acts; *per se* and in themselves they are not capable of being ordered to God and to the good of the person. "As for acts which are themselves sins [*cum iam opera ipsa peccata sunt*], Saint Augustine writes, like theft, fornication, blasphemy, who would dare affirm that, by doing them for good motives [*causis bonis*], they would no longer be sins, or, what is even more absurd, that they would be sins that are justified?" Consequently, circumstances or intentions can never transform an act intrinsically evil by virtue of its object into an act "subjectively" good or defensible as a choice.[20]

An intrinsically evil act should never be done, even for the most noble of purposes, such as securing heaven for someone.

Now a different question arises. Is abortion an intrinsically evil act? In the words of Pope St. John Paul II: "Given such unanimity in the doctrinal and disciplinary tradition of the Church, Paul VI was able to declare that this tradition is unchanged and unchangeable. Therefore, by the authority which Christ conferred upon Peter and his Successors, in communion with the Bishops—who on various occasions have condemned abortion and who in the aforementioned consultation, albeit dispersed throughout the world, have shown unanimous agreement concerning this doctrine— I declare that direct abortion, that is, abortion willed as an end or as a means, always constitutes a grave moral disorder, since it is the deliberate killing of an innocent human being."[21] Given this teaching, if we accept the Pauline Principle, Dan Thomas's case for a Pro-life Paradox collapses.

For the sake of argument, let us consider a theological consequentialist view that there is no such thing as an intrinsically evil act and that we should do whatever act maximizes the likelihood of salvation of the greatest number. Would it follow from this assumption that we should kill prenatal human beings so as to assure that they automatically get to heaven? Even given these (anti-)Christian presuppositions, an affirmative answer would be unwarranted. After all, consequentialism is not just about maximizing the good for one person but must concern itself with the greatest good for the greatest number of persons. Even if aborting a prenatal human being would assure that this one person obtains eternal salvation, it may still be wrong to kill him or her because it may not bring about the greatest good for the greatest number of people. Some people, such as St. Francis Xavier, Pope St. John Paul II, and St. Mother Teresa of Calcutta, cooperated with God to aid the salvation of many, many people. If any of these great saints had died prior to undertaking their important works of evangelization, the salvation of many other people would have been endangered. In contemplating killing a child prior to reason, we cannot exclude the possibility that we are depriving the world of a future great saint who would have aided in the salvation of many other people. So, even on the grounds of a consequentialism seeking to maximize the likelihood of salvation for the greatest number of people, the conclusion that Dan Thomas draws, given the Pro-life Paradox, is not justified.

Another problem with the Pro-life Paradox is that it assumes that the only good that really matters is the good of eternal life. From a Christian perspective, this supposition is false. Christians take the life and teachings of Jesus as their fundamental guide to what matters. But the example of Jesus suggests that Christ cares, not simply and only about the good of souls, but also about other goods. In healing the blind, Jesus's example points to the importance of vision. In raising the dead back to life, Christ underscores the value of terrestrial human life. In turning water into wine, the son of Mary emphasizes the importance of marriage and social celebration. Most of all, Jesus consistently cares for rather than kills the weak and vulnerable in his society, whether it is the woman caught in adultery, the Samaritan woman at the well, or the leper cast out of human community. In trying to secure that every human being is protected by law and welcomed in life, Christian prolife advocates are following the example of Jesus in caring for the vulnerable and defenseless.

Yet another problem with Dan Thomas's "Pro-life Paradox" is that Christians are called to love *all* human beings without exception, not just those who might be killed in abortion and then go to heaven. Abortionists have souls too, and Christians are called to care about their souls as well. Even if abortion were not intrinsically evil, it is clearly and obviously contrary to the teachings and disciplines of the Church. For this reason, Pope St. John Paul II notes in *Evangelium vitae*:

> The Church's canonical discipline, from the earliest centuries, has inflicted penal sanctions on those guilty of abortion. This practice, with

more or less severe penalties, has been confirmed in various periods of history. The 1917 Code of Canon Law punished abortion with excommunication. The revised canonical legislation continues this tradition when it decrees that "a person who actually procures an abortion incurs automatic [*latae sententiae*] excommunication." The excommunication affects all those who commit this crime with knowledge of the penalty attached, and thus includes those accomplices without whose help the crime would not have been committed. By this reiterated sanction, the Church makes clear that abortion is a most serious and dangerous crime, thereby encouraging those who commit it to seek without delay the path of conversion. In the Church the purpose of the penalty of excommunication is to make an individual fully aware of the gravity of a certain sin and then to foster genuine conversion and repentance.[22]

The penalty of excommunication is intended to stimulate repentance, to prompt a change of heart, and to lead to a reformation of life. In imitation of Jesus, Christians are called to love every human being, every sinner, and to work and pray for their salvation. To celebrate the work of abortionists is at cross-purposes with the call to help them live in harmony with God's church.

In sum, the "Pro-life Paradox" is no paradox if other fundamental Christian teachings are kept in mind. Against the teachings of Augustine, Aquinas, and the *Catechism of the Catholic Church*, the Pro-life Paradox presumes that all infants automatically go to heaven. Against the teaching of scripture and the Church, the Pro-life Paradox assumes that one may do evil so that good may come of it. Against the example and teaching of Jesus, the Pro-life Paradox implicitly assumes that the only good that matters is eternal life. The argument made by Dan Thomas shows no concern about the souls of abortionists who act in a way that incurs automatic excommunication from the Church. In sum, for anyone accepting any of these basic Christian teachings, the Pro-life Paradox is no problem at all.

Seven

Is There a Right to the Death of the Fetus?

THE ABORTION DEBATE APPEARS TO BE INTERMINABLE. BUT MAYBE there is hope that the debate will end. Both defenders and critics of abortion have taken up the question, "Could artificial wombs end the abortion debate?" If the prenatal human being, a member of the biological species *Homo sapiens*, could be removed from the uterus (ectogenesis), an unwanted pregnancy would be over. This outcome is pleasing to those who advocate for a woman's right to terminate her pregnancy. If the living prenatal human being was then placed in an advanced incubator (artificial womb), then no human being would die. This outcome is pleasing to those who advocate for the human right to live of prenatal human beings. The "win-win" scenario of providing artificial wombs rather than ending the life of the prenatal human being has been endorsed by a number of authors on all sides of the abortion debate.[1]

In his article "Abortion and a Right to the Death of the Fetus,"[2] Joona Räsänen challenges this view by providing three arguments for a right to secure the death of the human being in utero. On his view, abortion

61

includes the right to the death of the gestating human being, not merely a removal of the prenatal human being from the uterus.

THE RIGHT NOT TO BECOME A BIOLOGICAL PARENT ARGUMENT

First, Räsänen offers the Right Not to Become a Biological Parent Argument. He states it as follows:

1. Becoming a biological parent causes harm to the couple because of parental obligations towards the child.
2. The couple has the interest to avoid the harm of parental obligations.
3. Therefore, the couple has a right to the death of the fetus to avoid the harm of parental obligations.[3]

This argument is logically invalid. The phrase "a right to the death of the fetus" is in neither the major nor the minor premise, so it cannot appear like a rabbit out of a hat in the conclusion. So even if both premises were true, they would not provide a justification for the conclusion.

One could make new versions of the Right Not to Become a Biological Parent Argument by using either one of the two original premises. For example, one new valid version of the Right Not to Become a Biological Parent Argument could be stated as follows:

1. If the couple has the interest to avoid the harm of parental obligations, then the couple has a right to the death of the fetus to avoid the harm of parental obligations.
2. The couple has the interest to avoid the harm of parental obligations.
3. Therefore, the couple has a right to the death of the fetus to avoid the harm of parental obligations.

A similar reconstruction could be made from use of the other original premise, "Becoming a biological parent causes harm to the couple because of parental obligations towards the child." So let us consider both original premises. Does Räsänen give us good reason to think that both premises are true?

The reason given for the first premise, "Becoming a biological parent causes harm to the couple because of parental obligations towards the child," is that "parents would still feel morally responsible for the child, which then could cause them significant psychological harm."[4] This reason does not provide justification for the premise. To say something *could* cause harm does not show that something *does* cause harm.

Moreover, Räsänen provides no empirical evidence that becoming biological parents could cause the couple significant psychological harm. On the contrary, many people report that unplanned parenthood turned out to be not a curse but rather a great gift in their lives.[5] Almost all parents view their own children, whatever the circumstances of their conception, as an unambiguous blessing rather than as a harm.

But the case that Räsänen has in mind is not parents who raise their children who were conceived in unplanned ways but rather biological parents who place their children into another family via adoption. Would parents who place their children for adoption after ectogenesis experience psychological burdens from making that choice and knowing that their biological offspring was being raised by someone else?

It is difficult to answer this question because we have no empirical evidence about the psychological effects of currently nonexistent ectogenesis. Even if some birth mothers now experience trauma in placing a child for adoption, this would not show that *ectogenesis* leads to trauma. It could be that after nine months of pregnancy, psychological bonds develop such that adoption becomes traumatic. It could be that the social aspects of pregnancy, such as the knowledge of other people about a woman's pregnancy, make adoption at nine months difficult. If ectogenesis is used a short time after pregnancy is detected, there may not be sufficient time to develop such bonds or for the social aspects of pregnancy to be relevant. So it could turn out that full-term birth, but not ectogenesis, leads to trauma.

In fact, the evidence suggests that it is not becoming a biological parent but getting an abortion that can cause significant psychological harm. In several studies, David M. Fergusson, professor of psychology at the University of Otago, has noted that abortion itself is a risk factor for psychological harm.[6] Lest the credibility of these studies be called into question because it is assumed that this psychologist is prolife, Dr. Fergusson describes himself as prochoice.[7] Fergusson and colleagues concluded,

We have used extensive data gathered over the course of a 30-year longitudinal study to examine the links between a series of pregnancy
outcomes (abortion, pregnancy loss, unwanted pregnancy leading to
live birth, and other live birth) and common mental health outcomes,
including depression, anxiety, suicidal behaviours and substance use
disorders. The major finding of this analysis is that even following
extensive control for prospectively and concurrently measured con-
founders, women who had had abortions had rates of mental health
problems that were about *30% higher than rates of disorder in other
women*. Although rates of all forms of disorder were higher in women
exposed to abortion, the conditions most associated with abortion included anxiety disorders and substance use disorders. In contrast,
none of the other pregnancy outcomes (pregnancy loss, live birth following unwanted pregnancy or a pregnancy having an initial adverse
reaction, and other live birth) was consistently related to significantly
increased risks of mental health problems.[8]

So if we are focusing on avoiding the risk of substantial psychological
harm, it is not biological parenthood we should avoid but abortion.

Another problematic element of the Right Not to Become a Biological
Parent Argument is its internal inconsistency about parenthood. Räsänen
writes, "In this article, I use the terms genetic parent and biological parent
as synonyms."[9] He holds that "there is a right to the death of the fetus because gestating a fetus in an artificial womb when genetic parents refuse it
violates their rights not to become a biological parent."[10] But someone who
already is a biological parent cannot have the right not to become a biological parent. Rights have to do with choices that are possible. But someone who already *is* a biological parent to an individual cannot *become* a
biological parent to that individual. Once a human being has been conceived, the man and the woman have already become biological/genetic
parents, so the opportunity to exercise the putative right not to *become* a
genetic/biological parent has passed—that ship has sailed.

Someone might posit a right not to *remain* a biological parent, a modern *patria potestas*, but that is presumably a different kind of claim. It is
also hard to see how the right not to remain a biological parent can be
squared with the legal and ethical responsibilities that biological parents
are thought to have to their vulnerable, dependent children.

Indeed, it is plausible to hold that parental rights arise *because* of parental duties.[11] Parents cannot discharge their duties to care for and keep safe their children unless they have special rights to control their children that others do not have. For this reason, parents who fail in their parental duties (by endangering or even intentionally harming their children) sometimes have their parental rights terminated. If parental duties circumscribe and ground parental rights, parental rights cannot justify actions that contradict parental duties to care for and above all not harm vulnerable, dependent children.

THE RIGHT TO GENETIC PRIVACY ARGUMENT

Let us now consider the Right to Genetic Privacy Argument. In the following argument, by *ectogenesis abortion*, Räsänen means a doctor's removal of the living premature fetus from the uterus into an intensive care unit that will facilitate the continued life of the fetus. In the case envisioned, ectogenesis abortion would be done with prior authorization of the pregnant woman. Räsänen articulates this argument as follows:

1. People have a right to genetic privacy.
2. Ectogenesis abortion violates the genetic privacy of the genetic parents of the fetus.
3. Therefore, genetic parents have a right to the death of the fetus.[12]

This argument is logically invalid. The phrase "a right to the death of the fetus" does not appear in either of the premises but arrives via a non sequitur in the conclusion.

New versions of the Right to Genetic Privacy Argument could be made by use of either one of the two original premises. For example, we could revise the Right to Genetic Privacy Argument as follows:

1. If ectogenesis abortion violates the genetic privacy of the genetic parents of the fetus, then genetic parents have a right to the death of the fetus.
2. Ectogenesis abortion violates the genetic privacy of the genetic parents of the fetus.
3. Therefore, genetic parents have a right to the death of the fetus.

This new version of the Right to Genetic Privacy Argument is logically valid. We could construct another new version of the Right to Genetic Privacy argument making use of the other original premise, "People have a right to genetic privacy." The question then arises, are either of the original premises of the Right to Genetic Privacy Argument true?

An example given by Räsänen to illustrate a right to genetic privacy seems intuitively plausible to me. If someone steals my genetic material in order to make a clone of me and gestates that cloned individual via ectogenesis, that person wrongs me in a significant way. Räsänen takes a large step beyond this intuition, saying that "therefore, in such a case, I have a right to the death of the fetus."[13] But it does not follow from the premise that I have been wronged in the Stolen Genetic Material Case that I have a right to the death of the cloned individual. After all, suppose I found out that my genetic material had been stolen and I had been cloned ten years after the cloning took place. Surely, Räsänen does not believe that I would be justified in killing my fifth-grade clone. So it does not follow from the intuition that I have been wronged in the Stolen Genetic Material Case that I have a right to the death of an individual made from my stolen genetic material.

Moreover, our shared intuition about the Stolen Genetic Material Case justifies only the relatively weak claim that *in some cases* people have a right to genetic privacy. The Stolen Genetic Material Case does not show the stronger claim that *in all cases* people have a right to genetic privacy. But the Right to Genetic Privacy Argument needs the stronger claim. After all, *if* in some cases people have a right to genetic privacy and in some cases they do not, then it could be that ectogenesis is a case in which people do not have a right to genetic privacy. Räsänen has not provided any reason to think that the stronger claim is true.

Another difficulty with Räsänen's overall case for securing the death of the fetus is that the Right to Genetic Privacy Argument is incompatible with the Right Not to Become a Biological Parent Argument. One cannot consistently assert both arguments because the premises of these arguments are contradictory. The Right Not to Become a Biological Parent Argument is based on the premise that "becoming a biological parent causes harm to the couple because of parental obligations towards the child." The Right to Genetic Privacy Argument is based on the premise that "ectogenesis abortion violates the genetic privacy of the genetic parents of the fetus." Räsänen holds that women have their genetic privacy rights violated if their genetic children carry their genetic material without consent.

Recall that for Räsänen the terms *genetic parent* and *biological parent* are synonyms.[14] Therefore according to the first argument the man and woman in question are *not yet* biological parents, so they can kill the fetal human being to prevent themselves from becoming biological parents. In the second argument, the man and woman are *already* biological parents, so they can kill the fetal human being. Are the man and the woman biological or genetic parents of this prenatal son or daughter? If we answer affirmatively, the first argument fails. If we answer negatively, the second argument fails. But whether we answer affirmatively or negatively, the two arguments are incompatible with one another, for they embody contradictory understandings of when genetic/biological parenthood begins.

THE RIGHT TO PROPERTY ARGUMENT

A third argument, called The Right to Property Argument, Räsänen formulates as follows:

1. The fetus is property of the genetic parents.
2. People can destroy their property.
3. Therefore, genetic parents can destroy their fetus.[15]

This argument is logically invalid. Exemplifying the four-term fallacy, the Right to Property Argument is a categorical syllogism with more than three terms, namely "the fetus," "property of the genetic parents," "people," "can destroy their property," "genetic parents" and "can destroy their fetus." The Right to Property Argument also commits the fallacy of undistributed middle, since the middle term "property" is not distributed in Räsänen's formulation of the argument.[16]

A new version of the Right to Property Argument could be formulated as follows:

1. If the fetus is property of the genetic parents, the genetic parents may destroy their fetus.

2.   The fetus is property of the genetic parents.
3.   Therefore, genetic parents may destroy their fetus.

This version of the Right to Property Argument is logically valid. But are both premises of the revised Right to Property Argument true?

The second premise is deeply questionable. *Parent* is a relational term. There is no such thing as a parent without a child. If there is a human parent, there is also a human child. The relationship of parent to child is not the relationship of owner to property. For this reason, critics of abortion speak of the "unborn child" but defenders of abortion do not, for they (rightly) note that the term is question begging. The parent-child relationship is not a neutral, biological categorization but rather a morally loaded way of speaking of a relationship that suggests that the parents ought to provide for their vulnerable child. But if it is implicitly admitted that a child is present, then a crucial premise of the prolife argument is admitted. No human child is the property of another, and parents in particular owe their own dependent progeny treatment not as objects to be destroyed but as children to be cherished.

Moreover, the conclusion of the Right to Property Argument that "genetic parents may destroy their fetus" is at odds with Räsänen's assertion that "I have not argued that biological parents have a right to kill the fetus, but that they have a right to the death of the fetus."[17] It is physically (and perhaps also metaphysically) impossible for someone to destroy the fetus but not kill the fetus. So if Räsänen is right in his argument that genetic parents have a right to destroy their child, then Räsänen is wrong that he has not argued for a right to kill.

Not the mother alone and not the father alone have the right to kill their son or daughter. Räsänen writes: "I claim that the fetus is collective property of its genetic parents. When the genetic parents agree and they both want the death of the fetus or the destruction of the embryos, it is morally permissible for them to do so since they together share 100% of the fetus' or the embryos' genetic material, and gestating the fetus or the embryos against their consent violates their rights."[18] This grounding for a right to kill the fetus echoes his earlier claim that people have their right to genetic privacy violated in cases in which there are "genetic children out there who carry their genetic material without their consent."[19] Since both the mother and the father are the genetic parents, the right to genetic privacy is understood as a collective right rather than as an individual right. Räsänen writes, "100% of the fetus' genetic material comes from its genetic parents. Because having a genetic child in the world who carries the genetic material of the parents without their consent is against their right to genetic privacy, the genetic parents together have a right to the death of the fetus."[20] So, on his view, the mother alone or the father alone does not have a right to secure the death of his or her son or daughter but only both parents together.

Now, by parity of reasoning, it is equally true that 100 percent of the fetus's genetic material comes from his or her genetic grandparents. Because having a genetic grandchild in the world who carries the genetic material of the grandparents without their consent is against their right to genetic privacy, the genetic grandparents together have a right to the death of the fetus. This is hard to believe. So the fact that a child's genetic material comes 100 percent from some group of people is irrelevant to whether those people have a right, if they all agree, to the death of their child.

Finally, neither parents nor grandparents should consider their child or grandchild their genetic property. Epigenetic factors are essential to how any particular genotype is expressed. So an human individual has a uniquely expressed genotype that is *not* entirely derived from the parents or grandparents. Because of environmental factors, all human individuals (even those deriving from the same fertilized egg) have a unique expressed genotype.

CONCLUSION

In conclusion, all three of Räsänen's arguments for the conclusion that the parents have a right to the death of their son or daughter fail. The Right Not to Become a Biological Parent Argument, the Right to Genetic Privacy Argument, and the Right to Property Argument are all logically invalid. These arguments also make use of premises that are not consistent with each other. There is also reason to question whether all the premises of these arguments are true.[21]

Eight

Why Should the Baby Live?

ABORTION IS CONTROVERSIAL, BUT INFANTICIDE IS EVEN MORE controversial. Alberto Giubilini and Francesca Minerva's essay "After-birth Abortion: Why Should the Baby Live?" aroused more consternation than any other article in contemporary bioethics.[1] Giubilini and Minerva's view is that parents may intentionally kill their newborn, even if she is perfectly healthy and desired by others for adoption.

They come to this conclusion on the basis of their view that a "person" in the moral sense is properly defined as an individual who values her own existence. If a person is an individual who values her own existence (and therefore must as a precondition know of her own existence), both the newborn baby and the fetus are not actual persons but only potential persons. If both the prenatal fetus and a postnatal infant do not have a right to live, Giubilini and Minerva draw the conclusion that "when circumstances occur after birth such that they would have justified abortion, what we call after-birth abortion should be permissible."[2]

Since many advocates of abortion rights support abortion on demand, if Giubilini and Minerva's argument is sound, postbirth abortion on demand, even of perfectly healthy babies, is also permissible.

After the online publication of Alberto Giubilini and Francesca Minerva's article, there was an immediate and almost overwhelmingly negative reaction around the world. Their article was published in print in the May 2013 edition of the *Journal of Medical Ethics* alongside more than twenty reflections and reactions to it.

These essays, on the whole, are disappointing. For the most part, they rehash old arguments—in some cases arguments that were first put forward four decades ago. This is not altogether surprising, since Giubilini and Minerva's article recycles (in a less sophisticated form) Michael Tooley's defense of infanticide from 1972.[3]

One of the best of these essays is "Yes, the Baby Should Live: A Prochoice Response to Giubilini and Minerva," by Bertha Alvarez Manninen.[4] Manninen points out, quite rightly, that Giubilini and Minerva's view may even allow the killing of three-year-old children who do not in all cases fulfill Locke's definition of a person: "a thinking, intelligent being, that has reason and reflection, and can consider itself as itself, the same thinking thing, in different times, and places; which it does only by that consciousness which is inseparable from thinking, and, as it seems to me, essential to it."[5] Giubilini, Minerva, and Tooley surely are aware that their position entails the conclusion that children two or three years of age do not have a right to live. But they decline to state this implication explicitly, for this implication amounts (for most people) to a reductio ad absurdum of their position.

Locke's account of a person is aimed at answering the question: Which individuals can we hold ethically accountable for their actions? Locke is not using his account of personhood to answer the question: Who is to be accorded basic rights? It makes no sense to hold a human being accountable for his or her actions unless that individual is a source of responsibility. Without robust self-reflection and memory, a person cannot be a source of responsibility and held accountable for his or her actions. Yet if we hold that the right to live is tied to the ability to be a source of responsibility, then full moral status does not begin until the so-called "age of reason," customarily held to be seven years of age.

It is true that Giubilini and Minerva's account of what constitutes a person is less stringent than Locke's. Nevertheless, Manninen notes that "the mental traits they argue [are] a prerequisite to possessing a right to life do not appear overnight, and they are not lost instantaneously either. Is the right to life a gradient right? Does a 1-year-old have just a little bit of that right—less than a 5-year-old, but more than a neonate? If an elderly individual begins the degeneration into Alzheimer's disease, does her right to life become gradually weaker?"[6] This insight could be developed into what is sometimes called the equality argument. If our moral rights are based on degreed characteristics, then the more we have of a value-making characteristic, the greater the value we have and the greater the right to life we have. But this contradicts the widely held notion that all human persons have fundamentally equal rights. As John Finnis points out in his contribution, "The declarations of human equality (factual and moral) were solemnly reaffirmed after the sobering, thought-provoking experiences of the mid- 20th century. They are a better standard for confirmation of a critically philosophical argument about these matters than is provided by laws and conventions all too easily (but truly) explicable by reference to the self-interest of people who, relative to the human beings under discussion in Giubilini and Minerva's paper, are people of power."[7] Anyone concerned about vulnerable human populations surely must include defenseless, innocent babies.

Giubilini and Minerva deny that the newborn has equal rights because they hold that the neonate does not have an interest in living. Manninen, following Steinbock and others, denies this by distinguishing between two meanings of *interest*. A person has an objective interest in something (what Manninen calls "interest 1") and a subjective interest (what Manninen calls "interest 2").[8] Nonhuman animals have an objective interest in receiving vaccinations so that they do not get sick and die, but they do not have a subjective interest in such vaccinations because they do not know what "health" is, nor do they know the connections between vaccinations and health or envision what their life will be like if they do not get vaccinations. Similarly, Manninen points out that children who are mentally handicapped have an objective interest in becoming educated to a greater degree (interest 1) even though they may not subjectively be interested in getting an education (interest 2). Clearly, a human being can be benefited without appreciating it, caring about it, or even being aware of it. So too a human being can be harmed without appreciating it, caring about it, or even being aware of it. Benefit and harm are similar in that one makes an individual better off and the other makes an individual worse off, but having an interest 2 is not necessary to having an interest 1. Indeed, sometimes what a person is subjectively interested in gaining will actually be detrimental to what would be objectively good to have, such as drugs for an addict who desperately wants another fix and equally desperately wants to avoid rehabilitation.

Manninen's arguments from objective interests for attributing moral status to newborn human beings can also be applied to prenatal human beings. Unborn children too have an objective interest in living. Nevertheless, Manninen seeks to defend the conventional prochoice view that infanticide is impermissible but abortion is permissible. She does not hold that neonatal human beings and prenatal human beings late in pregnancy differ intrinsically in their moral status. Rather, she justifies her defense of abortion by a version of the Violinist Analogy (mentioned earlier in chapter 3 of this volume). She writes,

> No person (whether intrauterine or extrauterine) has a right to use the body of another for sustenance. In this sense, embryos and fetuses would be entitled to the same care and protection as any other person—while the vulnerable need care and protection, that protection can never extend to the point that the bodily autonomy of another may be violated. A sick patient in need of a bone marrow transplant, for example, should be cared for and protected as much as possible, and every avenue available to secure him a bone marrow transplant should be pursued. However, it would never be permissible to forcibly extract bone marrow from an unwilling "donor," and our refusal to do so is not typically interpreted as a refusal to care for the patient. Similarly, if it were possible to care for an embryo or fetus without encroaching on another person's bodily autonomy, then I would favour pursing that option and, if a fetus survives an abortion, then I do believe the infant should be given the same level of care and protection as any comparable newborn.[9]

According to this variation of the Violinist Analogy, Manninen concludes that "every person has a right to decide if they wish to use their body to sustain the life of another." I'm not sure this is true.

Imagine a father with his baby alone in a distant mountaintop cabin cut off from all forms of communication. At a certain point, the baby cries out for food, but the man is busy playing video games and says to himself, "To feed this hungry baby, I'd have to get up from my game, prepare a bottle, and then probably also hold the baby while she eats. I do not wish to use my body in this way. I have the right to decide if I wish to use my body to sustain another person. In doing this, I am doing nothing wrong whatsoever, since I am an autonomous person, and my body is free for me to use as I please." As the weekend passes, the baby repeatedly cries out for food, and the man repeatedly invokes his previously mentioned ethical rationalization. When his baby dies, do we really believe that the father of this child has done nothing wrong?

One retort might be that the father in staying with the baby in the cabin has implicitly agreed to take on the responsibility for caring for the baby. But we can change the scenario to account for this objection. The father was simply visiting the cabin, and the mother took off from the isolated cabin in the only car available and left the father and baby there alone before the father made any (implicit) agreement.

It may be retorted that pregnancy is much more difficult for a mother than setting aside a video game is for the father. But what is at issue is not the amount of sacrifice involved in continuing a pregnancy or in caring for a newborn. The amount of sacrifice will vary widely depending on the circumstances of the pregnancy and the circumstances of caring for a newborn. Some pregnancies will be much easier to continue than some cases of caring for neonates. In other cases, caring for a neonate will be much more difficult than continuing a pregnancy, especially since some women do not even realize that they are pregnant.[10] The example of the father playing video games and fatally neglecting his baby is meant to indicate that it is not true that parents have an absolute right to decide whether they will use their body to sustain the life of their own dependent child. Parents have moral (and often legal) duties to provide basic care for their dependent minor children, even if they must use their bodies to do so.

However, Manninen is right that it is wrong, seriously wrong, to forcibly extract bone marrow from an unwilling "donor." But this insight does not justify abortion. In fact, it leads to the condemnation of most abortions. In typical cases of abortion, the bodily integrity of a prenatal body is forcibly violated as the human being in utero is violently dismembered and torn limb by limb out of the uterus. If forcibly extracting bone marrow from a person who is able to survive the extraction is wrong, a fortiori lethal dismemberment of a person's entire body is wrong.

Nor is it accurate to characterize abortion as simply the mother withdrawing aid and declining to use her body to support another person. An abortion, at least as far as the abortionist is concerned, is aimed at causing the death of the human being in utero (usually by dismemberment), not merely separating him or her from his or her mother. (I use the gendered possessive pronoun intentionally, for a prenatal human being is a "him" or a "her" as much as a postnatal human being is). The criminal case of Kermit Gosnell was about botched abortions in which he failed to do what he had initially attempted to do. If he had successfully killed the prenatal children as he was attempting to do in the abortions, he would have never been convicted of killing postnatal children. Nor is abortion properly characterized as "terminating a pregnancy," for "selective reduction" of a pregnancy, in which one twin is killed while the other twin is allowed to live, does not terminate a pregnancy but is nevertheless a case of abortion. In sum, Manninen's arguments do not succeed in differentiating the killing of neonates from the killing of prenatal human beings.

Neil Levy argues that perhaps people have the intuition that neonates differ in moral status from prenatal human beings because "birth is a necessary condition for the acquisition of important psychological properties (together, perhaps, with the fact that birth correlates reasonably well with age)."[11] One difficulty with this suggestion is that while birth may be a necessary condition for acquiring important psychological properties, there are many other necessary conditions for acquiring important psychological properties, such as having someone physically care for the newborn, speaking with the growing child, and being a living member of a species that can have such mental properties. The question then arises why having *this* necessary condition grants increased moral status while having *these* other necessary conditions does not. Why is birth so important and not, for example, verbal communication? Surely, feral children have basic rights even though, because of their lack of the necessary condition of conversation, they have developed psychological properties no greater than other nonhuman animals.

In "Of Course the Baby Should Live: Against 'After-birth Abortion,'" Regina A. Rini argues that a neonatal human being and a prenatal human being have differing moral status because the former has aims and the latter does not:

> Specifically, the human being becomes biologically independent of its mother, in such a way that it begins to have aims that it did not before. In the womb, a fetus is essentially passive regarding its own needs, which are provided directly by the umbilical cord and uterine environment. A newborn infant, once its umbilical cord has been severed, must suddenly begin to breathe on its own, to process its own nutrients, to digest and excrete and seek out warmth. It must almost immediately begin responding to these needs, playing the tiniest role in their accomplishment through its grasping, suckling and crying. As I suggested in the last section, these needs, along with the means to accomplish them, are very plausibly understood as "aims," at least to a similar extent that animals and certain disabled adults have aims. Newborn infants have aims, but fetuses do not. Therefore, if the vulnerability of such aims to frustration is morally significant, then there is a morally relevant difference between a fetus and a newborn. (N1) is false, so the Natal and Prenatal Equivalence Arguments both fail.[12]

The argument may be interpreted in a number of ways. Is it the baby's grasping, suckling, and crying that make the significant difference? All these are sometimes done in utero prior to birth. Is it breathing on her own, processing her own nutrients, digesting, excreting, and seeking out warmth that make a baby girl have greater status than an unborn girl? It is hard to see why any of these things is morally important. Any rat or frog is capable of such activities, which are mere instincts rather than rationally chosen "aims." Nor is it true that all prenatal human beings lack "aims" in the primitive, instinctive sense.

As reported in *Scientific American*:

> Researchers at the University of Turin and the University of Parma in Italy used ultrasonography, a technique for imaging internal body structures, to track the motion of five pairs of twin fetuses in daily

20-minute sessions. As published in the October *PLoS ONE*, the scientists found that fetuses begin reaching toward their neighbors by the 14th week of gestation. Over the following weeks they reduced the number of movements toward themselves and instead reached more frequently toward their counterparts. By the 18th week they spent more time contacting their partners than themselves or the walls of the uterus. Almost 30 percent of their movements were directed toward their prenatal companions. These movements, such as stroking the head or back, lasted longer and were more accurate than self-directed actions, such as touching their own eyes or mouth. The results suggest that twin fetuses are aware of their counterparts in the womb, that they prefer to interact with them, and that they respond to them in special ways. Contact between them appeared to be planned—not an accidental outcome of spatial proximity, says study co-author Cristina Becchio of Turin.[13]

If this research is accurate, twins in utero have "aims" at least as much as newborns. So are we then to conclude, using Rini's line of argument, that abortion of an individual is permissible but abortion of twins is not? In "Abortion, Infanticide and Moral Context," Lindsey Porter attempts to differentiate between abortion and infanticide in the following way: "Where, when pregnant, the woman is in a unique and singular sort of a relation with the fetus, such that it makes perfect sense to say that the choice is hers, this is simply not so once the newborn is outside her body. The baby is then—almost always—in various sorts of relationships with several or even many people. And where two progenitors are involved with a birth, the relationship between the woman and the baby is not even unique: the would-be father stands in the same potential-care-relation to the newborn that the would-be mother does."[14]

This analysis does not, in fact, distinguish all cases of abortion from all cases of infanticide. As just noted, prenatal twins are in a relationship with each other, yet presumably this does not change the permissibility of aborting twins. In some cases of (potential) infanticide, the woman is in a singular unique relationship with the baby. I am thinking of all cases in which a woman gives birth alone. She, and she alone, actually has a relationship with the newborn child such that she and she alone can care for that child. Furthermore, why does it make a difference to the moral status of a human being that the unique bodily relationship of the pregnant mother and her child is ended at birth? Indeed, once born, the infant is able to negatively impinge on the interests of more people.

Only after birth would a baby disturb others, cause economic hardship, and strain the requirements of sleep of not just one person but many. So if the interests of one actual person outweigh the interests of a potential person (the baby on Giubilini and Minerva's view), how much more would the interests of many actual persons outweigh the interest of one potential person. Reflections in the recent literature suggest the following conclusion: the arguments given against infanticide typically also undermine abortion; the arguments for abortion typically justify infanticide.

A CASE AGAINST OBJECTIONS TO INFANTICIDE

My book *The Ethics of Abortion: Women's Rights, Human Life, and the Question of Justice* offers four objections to Giubilini and Minerva's argument for infanticide.[15] First, they argue from deeply controversial cases to even more controversial conclusions. Second, they implicitly assume the truth of body-self dualism. Third, they cannot account for the equality of all persons. Finally, they assume a problematic account of what constitutes harm. Joona Räsänen, in his article "Pro-life Arguments against Infanticide and Why They Are Not Convincing," raises four critiques to these objections.[16] I will conclude this chapter by responding to his four critiques.

A First Objection against Infanticide: Arguing from the Controversial to the Even More Controversial

A first objection to Giubilini and Minerva's case for infanticide found in *The Ethics of Abortion* suggests that it is rhetorically dubious to appeal to deeply controversial premises to argue for what is even more controversial. For example, it is deeply controversial to assume that George W. Bush's invasion of Iraq was a just war. So it is problematic to assume "The Iraq War was just" as a premise for an even more controversial conclusion that the United States should now invade Iran. Giubilini and Minerva assume the permissibility of prebirth abortion, lethal embryo research, and capital punishment in their defense of postbirth abortion. But prebirth abortion, lethal embryo research, and capital punishment are among the most controversial ethical issues in contemporary society. So Giubilini and Minerva move from deeply controversial ethical positions to argue for an even more deeply controversial conclusion.

Räsänen answers this objection by saying, "Giubilini and Minerva think that some members of the human species do not have a right to life, but the reason for that is not the fact that capital punishment, abortion and embryo research are legal somewhere and that some people see those as morally acceptable practices but rather that not all human beings are persons who are capable of valuing their own existence."[17] These practices are mere illustrations of Giubilini and Minerva's underlying ethical principle that to be a person is to value your own continued existence. On Räsänen's view, these examples are simply conclusions following from the more general premise that only persons have a right to life.

While it is true that human beings who are killed in abortion or embryonic stem cell research do not value their own existence, Räsänen's defense fails to account for Giubilini and Minerva's inclusion of capital punishment in their list of morally acceptable practices. Most people sentenced to the death penalty value their own existence, and no one denies that human beings condemned to capital punishment are persons in the full moral sense. So Giubilini and Minerva's inclusion of the death penalty makes clear that they are not simply illustrating the principle that persons are individuals who value their own existence.

Moreover, the permissibility of prebirth abortion, lethal embryo research, and capital punishment does not necessarily presuppose a denial of the right to life to some human beings. Famously Judith Jarvis Thomson argues via the Violinist Analogy that abortion may be justified even if the human being in utero has a right to live because women have no obligation to keep the human fetus alive.[18] Likewise, John Finnis has defended the death penalty as an act of retributive justice that does not deny basic human rights to the condemned person.[19] If we understand the right to live as the right of innocent human beings not to be intentionally killed, then capital punishment (as well as killing in self-defense and killing enemy combatants in a just war) does not violate human rights. Jeff Mc-

Mahan argues that prior to implantation the human embryo is not sufficiently unified to be an organism.[20] If McMahan is right, then embryonic stem cell research that kills embryos is consistent with the principle of universal human rights for all human beings, since these embryos are not human beings. I do not believe Thomson or McMahan are in the end right, but their arguments do show that the premise of equal human rights for all human beings does not lead necessarily and without further argumentation to the conclusion that capital punishment, abortion, and embryo research are impermissible.

Importantly, none of these considerations justify intentionally killing a newborn baby. The Violinist Analogy does not apply because an infant does not depend upon her mother's body. Justifications of the death penalty are also irrelevant because no baby is justly convicted of a capital crime. Just war and killing in self-defense cannot justify infanticide because a baby is not a violent threat to anyone. And although some have called into question whether an embryo prior to implantation is an organism (and hence a human being), the claim that a newborn baby is not an organism is absurd.

A Second Objection against Infanticide: The Implausibility of Body-Self Dualism

A second objection raised in *The Ethics of Abortion* against infanticide calls into question Giubilini and Minerva's implicit body-self dualism. On this view, "you" are not a human being, a bodily organism of the human species. Properly speaking, "you" are your thoughts, ideas, desires, plans, and memories. So since your thoughts, ideas, desires, plans, and memories do not arise until months after birth, only at that point (around age two) did you, an individual who values her own existence, and therefore has a right to live, come into existence.

The Ethics of Abortion critiques body-self dualism as leading to absurd conclusions such as that you were never born, you have never seen yourself, and you have never been kissed. To kiss something involves bodily contact between the lips (one material thing) and something that receives the kiss (the other material thing). So if "you" are really your thoughts, ideas, desires, plans, and memories, these mental entities are not material (bodily) entities capable of being kissed. Moreover, consider the case of Dr. Robert Oxnam, who taught at Columbia University and is a former president of the Asian Society of New York. Oxnam suffers from a medical condition once called split personality disorder and now called dissociative identity disorder. Robert had eleven "alters," eleven independent sets of thoughts, ideas, desires, plans, and memories. Through much psychiatric intervention, he now has only three sets. If body-self dualism were true, then there would not be multiple *personalities* but multiple *persons* all inhabiting Robert's single human body. The psychiatrists who helped Robert to achieve greater psychological unity are would be in fact mass murderers who killed at least eight persons. This is hard to believe.

Räsänen does not deny that Giubilini and Minerva's defense of infanticide presupposes body-self dualism. Nor does Räsänen attempt to respond to these challenges or other challenges to body-self dualism.[21] Rather, Räsänen seeks to show that one alternative to body-self dualism, the Substance View (namely, that we are living bodily, animal organisms), is less plausible than body-self dualism because the Substance View entails the absurd view that abortion, infanticide, and killing an adult are all equally wrong. Räsänen's response exemplifies the *tu quoque* fallacy. If you are accused of theft, it does nothing to clear your name to claim that your accuser has also stolen.

Moreover, the presupposition of Räsänen's response is mistaken. According to Räsänen, the Substance View commits a person to the implausible view that early abortion, later abortion, infanticide, and killing a normal adult are all of equal moral gravity. *The Ethics of Abortion* treats this difficulty at length.[22]

To summarize quickly, according to a prolife perspective, all intentional killings of innocent human beings are alike in violating someone's right to live, but it is not true that all violations of the right to life are of equal moral gravity in all respects. Later abortion is normally more serious than early abortion for five reasons. First, in early abortion, the prenatal human being can experience no pain. In abortion just prior to birth, the prenatal human being can experience pain. To kill someone in a painful way adds an additional gravity to a killing.

Second, in early abortion, the burden of pregnancy has not yet been endured through the second and third trimester. By contrast, in a late-term abortion, most of the pregnancy has been completed, so it is (relatively) easier to finish the pregnancy. To fail to discharge a duty that is (relatively) easier to do is worse than to fail to discharge a duty that is (relatively) more difficult to do. Third, early in pregnancy, the humanity of the prenatal human being is more easily not understood. Just prior to birth, it is obvious to virtually everyone that the individual in question is alive and human. The culpability of an agent is in part determined by the knowledge of the agent. Early in pregnancy, it is more likely that an agent has inculpable ignorance about the humanity of the prenatal human being than later in pregnancy. Finally, in comparison to early abortion, late-term abortion has additional physical and emotional risks for the one getting the abortion.[23] The second, third, and fourth factors just mentioned also account for why infanticide is more seriously wrong than abortion. Killing an adult is worse than killing a newborn in terms of thwarting the plans of the individual, among other reasons.[24] There is no inconsistency in holding both that all innocent human beings have an equal right to life and that circumstances can make some violations of the right to live significantly worse than other violations. Indeed, all murders of adults are equally violations of their right to live, but both the civil law and common sense recognize aggravating circumstances making some murders worse than others, such as a criminal who murders the judge who sentenced him or a hit man who murders for money. The Substance View implies that all murders are equally wrong in terms of violating the right to life of the victim; the Substance View does not imply a blindness to aggravating or mitigating circumstances.

In another critique of the Substance View (SV), Räsänen writes, "In addition, if you or I came to be at conception (as supporters of SV claim), one might ask why we celebrate birthdays instead of conception days? After all, what is morally relevant, according to the supporters of SV, is the conception. But it would be ludicrous to celebrate the day you were conceived or count the years and days of how old you are from the date of the conception (at least as ludicrous than say that you or I were never born)."[25] We celebrate birthdays rather than conception days, so on Räsänen's view, it follows that the Substance View is mistaken. In other words, if the Substance View were right, we would celebrate days of conception rather than birthdays.

How might a defender of the Substance View respond? In some cultures, such as parts of Japan, age *is* calculated from conception. Why should we assume that the ways of our culture are superior to the ways of these cultures? Are we to say that the Substance View is true in such cultures but not true in those that do not celebrate conception? Does the permissibility of infanticide depend on geography? In fact, the Substance View and body-self dualism are both metaphysical accounts of human identity, and neither view depends upon cultural recognition. They are true or false regardless of cultural practice.

Moreover, it makes more sense to count age from birth than from conception for two reasons. The first is that a day of conception will often be hard to determine. Say a baby is born on July 15. If the child is not born prematurely, the baby was conceived sometime in October. But many couples do not keep careful track of the days on which they have sex, which makes finding a date of conception difficult. Even if they had intercourse only once and know the date, it would still not be clear on which day the child was conceived. Sperm can fertilize an egg up to five days after intercourse. A birth on July 15 is compatible with a wide range of dates, any of which is possible and none of which can be determined. It also makes sense to mark age from birth because birth (typically at least) is a more memorable, dramatic, and public event than conception. There is no inconsistency in celebrating birthdays and embracing the Substance View.

Räsänen offers another critique of the Substance View: "According to SV, we should let a 10-year-old boy die in a burning building and save, let's say, 10 frozen human embryos instead, if we were in a situation where we can save either the boy or the embryos. It would surely be better to save 10 valuable human beings than just one, so the rescuer should save the embryos rather than the boy. But this seems at least as odd a conclusion as accepting infanticide."[26] The embryo rescue case indicates that we should give up either the view that we are animal organisms or the idea that all human beings have a right to life. In other words, according to Räsänen, the Embryo Rescue Case shows that the Substance View is false.

The Ethics of Abortion claims that all human beings have equal basic value but also that some human beings may be more valuable than other human beings in other respects, such as desires to continue living, relationships with others, and responsibilities in the community.[27] These differences are relevant for the embryo rescue case. Räsänen is correct that some of these differences are extrinsic to the person (extrinsic in the sense of depending upon other people), such as responsibilities to other people, but Räsänen fails to notice that some of these aspects are intrinsic (within the person herself), like thwarted plans.

Furthermore, if someone rescues a ten-year-old boy, it is highly likely that he will live a normal life. But innumerable frozen embryos are never implanted, or do not survive the process of thawing and implantation, or spontaneously abort after implantation. In cases of triage, factors such as likelihood of survival are highly relevant to the question of who should be saved. Such factors make rescuing the ten-year-old, rather than ten embryos, permissible.

Moreover, the rescue case is irrelevant in terms of the right to life, which is properly understood as the right not to be intentionally killed, not the right to be rescued. The principles governing triage in rescue cases are not the same as the principles governing which human beings should be intentionally killed. It is not permissible to murder ten regular people in order to save a president or prime minister. However, if we cannot save them all, it is permissible to rescue a prime minster or president from death and to allow ten regular people to die in virtue of the special role of a world leader in the community. Similarly, it is at least permissible to save a ten-year-old boy and to allow ten embryos to die in virtue of the special role the boy has in the community with his friends, family, the investments already made in him by teachers and family, as well as his plans for his future. There is no inconsistency affirming equal basic rights for all human beings and rescuing a ten-year-old boy rather than ten frozen embryos.

Räsänen considers another explanation of why it is permissible to rescue the ten-year-old boy rather than ten frozen embryos:

> Friberg-Fernros states that although both the embryo and the child have an equal right to life, one should rescue the child because he has stronger time-relative interests than the embryo has. What he says is based on Jeff McMahan's Time-Relative Interest Account (TRIA). According to Friberg-Fernros, those stronger time-relative interests bring additional evil to the killing of the child compared with the killing

of the embryo and thus make the former worse. But this additional evil is just another way to say that the child has more intrinsic value than the embryo has—after all that additional evil is not like in the case of the president where killing has a negative impact on other people's lives.[28]

Here Räsänen misconstrues the argument. To claim that killing someone involves an additional evil is not just another way to say that the child has more intrinsic value than the embryo has. Yes, the additional evil in this case is not like that in the case of the president, where killing has a negative impact on other people's lives. But other sorts of additional evils might be in play. For example, all killing of innocent persons is intrinsically wrong, but for someone to murder his own mother involves an additional evil, since he owes his own mother a special love and honor. The claim that matricide is an additional evil to murder is not the claim that mothers have more intrinsic value than nonmothers. Similarly, the human embryo, the human fetus, the human baby, the human ten-year-old, and the human adult have equal basic intrinsic value as innate. But circumstantial considerations can make the killing of the human embryo different in certain morally relevant respects from the killing of the human fetus or a human baby. Likewise, circumstantial considerations can make the killing of a human ten-year-old circumstantially worse than killing a human baby. Only older human beings have time-relative interests in survival, and on that basis they might deserve to be rescued more than frozen embryos. To draw such distinctions is perfectly consistent with insisting upon the equal basic innate value of all human beings.

For the sake of argument, let's say all these defenses of the Substance View fail. Even if Räsänen is correct that body-self dualism is more problematic than the Substance View, it does not follow that Räsänen has provided an adequate defense of Giubilini and Minerva's view. The *tu quoque* fallacy makes clear that someone accused of theft does nothing to show his innocence by alleging that another person has stolen even more. Räsänen does not even attempt to respond to the objections raised against body-self dualism. So even if the Substance View were even more implausible than body-self dualism, this would do nothing to vindicate body-self dualism. After all, body-self dualism and the Substance View are not the only two options in debates about personal identity, so some third view (compatible with condemning infanticide) may be correct. To the extent that body-self dualism is implausible, Giubilini and Minerva's advocacy of infanticide is undermined.

A Third Objection against Infanticide: Equal Moral Worth

A third objection to Giubilini and Minerva's view is that all human persons have equal basic moral worth so that their worth cannot be based on a characteristic that comes in degrees. We do not all value our own lives to the same degree. Some people eat kale every morning for breakfast, walk an hour a day, and drink a glass of red wine with each dinner. Some people snort coke every morning, exercise only when evading law enforcement or other drug dealers, and enjoy racing cars on freeways while drunk on tequila. If what makes us valuable as persons is valuing our own lives, and we do not equally value our own lives, we do not all have equal value as persons.

On the contrary, contends Räsänen, we can hold both that the characteristic that makes someone a person comes in degrees and that all persons have equal value. Let's say that to be admitted to Princeton University requires a 4.4 grade point average. A grade point average is a degreed characteristic. Students admitted to Princeton are equally accepted students whether they barely passed the 4.4 threshold or whether they were admitted at the top of the class. So too, personhood is a based on a degreed characteristic, but once an individual gets over a certain threshold, that individual is admitted to the class of persons, enjoying equal rights with all other persons.

A classic challenge to the view that personhood is a threshold concept is the arbitrariness of choosing to draw the line in one place rather than another. In matters of life and death, we should not subject human beings to arbitrary line drawing. If an IQ of 40 does not get us beyond the threshold of personhood, why should an IQ of 41? How can a minuscule difference in intelligence justify intentionally killing one human being but provide the other human with the maximal moral protection of basic rights?

Räsänen answers this challenge to the threshold view of personhood by saying: "We don't need to actually choose or find that threshold, it is enough that we recognize that some beings (like fetuses and infants) are not even close to that threshold and others (normal human adults) are clearly beyond that threshold."[29] But if we don't actually choose a threshold or define what that threshold is, how can we know that an infant (or a fetus or a five-year-old) falls below it? If we don't choose or find a threshold, in virtue of what standard do "we know that fetuses and infants clearly are not persons even though it is difficult to determine when exactly a human being becomes a person"? Precisely at issue is whether the human infant is a person. The threshold concept of personhood is, in principle, neutral with respect to the question of the right to life of a baby because the threshold could be defined in a wide variety of ways (a beating heart, sentience, any brain activity, birth, valuing one's own existence, etc.). So we cannot know that no baby is a person unless we know what the threshold is and whether this threshold is justified.

Moreover, it is unjust to treat people in radically different ways because of insignificant differences. Räsänen points out that just a few points' difference on an entrance exam differentiates getting into a university with the full rights of a student as opposed to being rejected. True enough, but the difference between the case of admittance to a university and the case of infanticide is enormous. The penalty for not getting into Princeton is disappointment, not lethal injection. A Princeton reject may feel that his life is over, but an infant killed really has lost her life. To judge who is admitted to college admissions with threshold standards makes sense; to judge who is killed does not.

Moreover, meeting the performance threshold for academic admission is unlike meeting the performance threshold for having a right to live. In standards for academic admission, a university acting justly admits students in a nonarbitrary way by accepting only properly prepared students. Test scores, letters, and GPAs are admittedly imperfect measures of such preparation, but they characteristically have a real relationship to the ability to flourish academically. On the other hand, if the general argument of *The Ethics of Abortion* is correct, there is no rational basis for determining *which* degreed characteristic grants personhood (self-awareness, reasoning ability, communication skills, or sentience?) and *what degree* of that characteristic puts an individual over the threshold.

A Fourth Objection against Infanticide: Murder as Harm

A fourth objection against Giubulini and Minerva critiques their understanding of harm. On their view, in order for an individual to be harmed, it is necessary that the individual be "at least *in the condition* to value the different situation she would have found herself in if she had not been harmed."[30] Since a newborn baby is not in the condition to value anything, she cannot be harmed, even in getting killed.

A challenge to this view is that this understanding of harm cannot explain why the victim of a surprise, painless killing has been harmed. A sleeping politician who is shot in her head and dies immediately does not experience her death as a loss. Unless we assume the survival of consciousness in the dead (which advocates of infanticide characteristically reject), murder victims have no conscientious awareness and so do not value anything whatsoever, including valuing the different situation they would have found themselves in if they had not been killed. So if it is necessary for an individual to be "at least in the condition to value the different situation she would have found herself in if she had not been harmed" in order to be harmed, the politician assassinated in her sleep has not been harmed. This is hard to believe.

Räsänen responds to this challenge by noting, "We harm living person [*sic*] because she is in a condition to value different situations before that harm occurs, not after. If someone commits a murder and before that murder occurs the victim is in a condition to value not being murdered over being murdered, then she is harmed and so murder is morally impermissible."[31] The sleeping politician prior to getting killed values her life and so is harmed in losing her life, even though after she loses her life she does not experience that loss as a harm.

We can distinguish the *after-harm principle* from the *before-harm principle*. Räsänen does not defend the after-harm principle articulated by Giubulini and Minerva; rather, he introduces a new, different principle, the before-harm principle. The after-harm principle of Giubulini and Minerva considers the condition of the individual after the harm has occurred, and this version is vulnerable to the surprise, painless murder objection, for the victim is not in the condition to value the different situation she would have found herself in if she had not been harmed. The before-harm principle of Räsänen considers the condition of the individual before the harm has occurred, and it is not as vulnerable to the surprise, painless murder objection.

But the before-harm principle also leads to counterintuitive results, as the Baby Lobotomy Case shows. Let's say a lobotomy is given to a healthy newborn baby girl in order to more easily force her later into child prostitution and sex slavery. The lobotomy renders her seriously mentally handicapped for the rest of her life, and she always remains just shy of the threshold needed to count as a "person" in Giubilini and Minerva's sense. So her being forced into child prostitution does not violate the rights of a person. Even as a twenty-year-old adult, because of the severity of her mental handicap, she is never able to appreciate the state that she would have been in if she had not been lobotomized. Although the woman was never in a condition to value not being lobotomized over being lobotomized, it is very hard to believe that deliberately making her severely mentally handicapped did not harm her. Like the after-harm principle, the before-harm principle does not explain the harm that obviously occurs in the Baby Lobotomy Case. If both versions of the harm principle are implausible, neither version serves to justify infanticide.

CONCLUSION

J. Räsänen defends Giubilini and Minerva against four objections raised to their case for infanticide. This chapter argues that this defense fails. First, although those killed in abortion or stem cell research do not value their own existence, those killed in the death penalty do value their own existence. So it is not the case that the three examples used by Giubilini and Minerva simply illustrate the implications of their claim that persons are individuals who value their own existence. Moreover, even supposing that that abortion, stem cell research, and capital punishment are acceptable, it does not necessarily follow that all human beings are not persons. If Thomson, Finnis, and McMahan adequately defend abortion, capital punishment, and stem cell research, approval of these practices is compatible with affirming universal human rights. Second, the Substance

View does not have the counterintuitive implications claimed. Even if Räsänen is right that the Substance View is more problematic than body-self dualism, some third account of personal identity (compatible with condemning infanticide) may be correct. Räsänen commits the *tu quoque* fallacy arguing against the Substance View rather than defending body-self dualism from criticisms. The third criticism raised by Räsänen fails because the case of killing a newborn is not similar to the case of not letting a high school student into college. Finally, the fourth criticism does not succeed because Räsänen's alternative to the harm principle offered by Giubilini and Minerva fails to account for the harm of lobotomizing a newborn. In sum, Räsänen's defense of after-birth abortion does not succeed.

Nine

Do Children Have a Right to Be Loved?

SCHOLARS HAVE RECENTLY TURNED THEIR ATTENTION TO THE SUBJECT of children, specifically our duties toward them, including questions about their adoption. Mhairi Cowden's article "What's Love Got to Do with It? Why a Child Does Not Have a Right to Be Loved" critiques the view of Matthew Liao that children have a right to be loved.[1] Liao's justification for his view draws on empirical research about what is necessary for the flourishing of children, where flourishing is understood in terms of physical, emotional, and social well-being. After reviewing the empirical literature, Liao concludes that children have a right to be loved since children have a right to what is necessary for their flourishing, and it is necessary for the flourishing of children that they be loved by a parent or guardian. Cowden calls into question Liao's conclusion by challenging both the empirical justification for the claim that love is necessary for the flourishing of children and also the very idea that love (at least as it involves emotions) can be commanded.

One aspect of Cowden's strategy admits that children need sufficient human interaction, physical and psychological proximity to adults, and experiential stimulation to mature into well-adjusted adults. What she denies, however, is that these things are simply the same as "love." That is, one could imagine cases where a child received sufficient human interaction, physical and psychological proximity to adults, and experiential stimulation but was not loved, and the empirical question would then constitute whether treatment undermined the well-being of the child.

This objection raises one of the most ancient and important questions in philosophy: What is love? In the *Symposium*, the Platonic Socrates explored this question (at least as it relates to *eros*), and the exploration has continued to the present day. One response to Cowden's objection is to claim that "love" is just (positive) human interaction, proximity, and experiential stimulation of the proper kind. Indeed, today not just philosophers but also psychologists explore the nature of love. In her book *Love 2.0: How Our Supreme Emotion Affects Everything We Feel, Think, Do, and Become*, the positive psychologist Barbara Fredrickson defined love as "the momentary upwelling of three tightly interwoven events: first, a sharing of one or more positive emotions between you and another; second, a synchrony between your and the other person's biochemistry and behaviors; and third, a reflected motive to invest in each other's well-being that brings mutual care."[2] According to this definition, love necessarily includes some aspects of what Liao was talking about, specifically the emphasis on proximity and care. And yet, this definition is obviously not the only possible understanding of love. For Christians, in fact, Fredrickson's definition is somewhat problematic insofar as it assumes that love, to be really love, must always be mutual. But in the view of Jesus, we can love those who do not love us in return. We can and should love our enemies (Matt. 5:43–48).

As so many Socratic dialogues make clear, to define something is difficult, and at least part of the dispute between Cowden and Liao is about how to define love. When disagreeing about a definition, one strategy is to show that a rival definition is too narrow: it excludes an instance that clearly should count within the definition. Another strategy is to try to show that a definition is too broad, including things that clearly do not fall under the definition.

Liao characterizes parental love in the following way: "To love a child is to seek a highly intense interaction with the child, where one values the child for the child's sake, where one seeks to bring about and to maintain physical and psychological proximity with the child, where one seeks to promote the child's well-being for the child's sake, and where one desires that the child reciprocate or, at least, is responsive to, one's love."[3] Cowden does not offer a rival definition of love. She focuses rather on ways in which Liao's characterization of love fails insofar as it is too broad in some respects and too narrow in others. It is too broad because many things that are typically connected to love, such as beneficial treatment, may not in every instance include love. Imagine a racist criminal forced to serve people of color at their lunchtime meal who hates those he serves but nevertheless provides a beneficial service. Here the benefit is present, but love is absent. Cowden objects that Liao's definition may also be too narrow because love may also lead to adverse treatment when combined with ignorance of specifics or because the emotions involved lead to distortions in treatment. A mother inspired by love gives her child aspirin to relieve his pain, not realizing that aspirin may cause potentially fatal Reye's syndrome. A loving father becomes overly protective of his daughter, hindering her social growth, precisely because of his deep love for her. In these cases, love is present, but benefit is absent.

Liao responds to Cowden's article directly and to my mind convincingly.[4] Part of his response is to challenge Cowden's empirical claims in part by suggesting that the best available empirical research does suggest that children need to experience loving actions from caring adults in order to fully flourish as adults. One response to the claim of Liao's definition of love being overinclusive and underinclusive is to distinguish between what a person who loves intends to do, proximately and remotely, and what actually results from the actions of the person who loves. The mother who mistakenly gives her child aspirin may truly be inspired by love, despite the fact that rather than benefiting the child, she in fact harms her child. A person who loves always *aims at* securing the good of the beloved, but the benevolent aims of a loving person can and do fail for a variety of reasons.

This brings us back to the question of how to define love. The best understanding of love (parental, erotic, friendly) of which I am aware is provided by Alexander Pruss in his brilliant book *One Body: An Essay on*

Christian Sexual Ethics.[5] On Pruss's view, love is not just doing good things: it includes appreciation of the one we love and the pursuit of unity in appropriate ways with the one we love. The racist criminal mentioned earlier is lacking both these elements. He does not appreciate the good in those he serves, he does not want to be united with them, and he is united with them only under compulsion, so that his will is not freely united with them. The criminal, then, is not really loving despite having one of the elements of love—beneficial action. If we adopt Pruss's definition, then the problem suggested by Cowden disappears.

That parents should love their children is not as controversial an assertion as the claim that people who wish to become parents have a duty to pursue this desire only by adoption rather than by procreation. In their article "The Bad Habit of Bearing Children," Heleana Theixos and S. B. Jamil scrutinize the choice to procreate and raise biological children and argue that adults who desire children should adopt children rather than have their own biological children.[6] Many premises of Theixos and Jamil's argument are well established, such as that orphans (defined by them as children without a primary caregiver) characteristically suffer mental, social, and physical problems both in the short term and in the long term to a much greater degree than nonorphans. The second premise of their argument is that we also have a serious (but defeasible) obligation to care for those who are in need. They appeal to Peter Singer's formulation of this obligation: "If it is in our power to prevent something bad from happening, without thereby sacrificing something of comparable moral importance, we ought, morally, to do it. . . . [This principle] requires us only to prevent what is bad, and not to promote what is good, and it requires this of us only when we can do it without sacrificing anything that is, from the moral point of view, comparably important."[7] The conclusion they draw is that those who desire to be parents often have a serious obligation to adopt existing orphans rather than have their own biological children. The authors criticize what they call "bionormativity," namely, the presumption that the biological bonds created by procreation are superior to other ways to form families, such as via adoption.

A key but relatively unexplored aspect of their argument is the relationship between duty and desire. On the one hand, the desire to be a biological parent, to experience pregnancy and childbirth, and to nurse one's own biological offspring is, on Theixos and Jamil's view, not so important as to justify forgoing the adoption of an orphan in favor of natural procreation. On the other hand, a person who does not desire to become a parent has no obligation to adopt an orphan precisely because of a lack of desire to be a parent. Now, for some people, the desire not to be a parent might be quite weak. Such persons may have no positive desire to be parents, but if it "happened" they would not be very upset at all. On the other hand, other people have extremely strong desires not just to be parents but to be biological parents. These intense desires to be biological parents lead some people to spend thousands and thousands of dollars on in vitro fertilization, to undergo painful and intrusive medical procedures, and to seek out the challenges of pregnancy.

Theixos and Jamil also hold that the onerous paperwork, time, financial cost, and hassles of adoption defeat the obligation to rescue orphans. Unfortunately, they are correct that adoption often involves a troublesomely difficult process. But surely the difficulties of the process of adoption, given its lamentable expenses and hassles, are not morally comparable to the sufferings of unadopted orphans. Given the choice between allowing a child to remain an orphan and going through the hassles of adoption, no reasonable person behind a Rawlsian veil of ignorance would choose to let a child remain an orphan, since the short-term and long-term difficulties of a child with no caregiver vastly outweigh those of the adoption process.

In a response to Theixos and Jamil's article, Karey Horwood, in "Bad Habit or Considered Decision," considers whether perhaps Theixos and Jamil have underestimated the importance of "bionormativity." She writes,

> No doubt all of us absorb messages about the "superiority" of biological procreation, just as we absorb heteronormative messages about the necessity of having one mother and one father, and just as we absorb messages that children must be raised in a family with two parents rather than in a communal setting. All of these normative ideals could be equally arbitrary and indefensible. Or maybe some of them, upon closer examination, might hold up to scrutiny. The point is that without digging deeply into the particulars to ferret out the difference between mere habit (or even prejudice) and a well-considered

conviction about the basis of human flourishing, there is no place from which to stand and judge with confidence that "all preferences that can be formulated as based on conceptions of parenting rooted in bionormative values cannot override the orphan's claim to rescue."[8]

What differences, if any, exist on average between children raised by their own biological parents and children raised by parents who adopted them? This is an interesting empirical question, but one that I will not now pursue further.

Another aspect of the subject of adoption is embryo adoption.[9] Thomas Nelson's article "Personhood and Embryo Adoption" defends the thesis that heterologous embryo transfer for rescue (HETr), the transfer of a human embryo to a woman who is not biologically the mother of the embryo, is morally impermissible. He notes that opponents of HETr often argue that the procreative good includes not just conception of a human being but also the nurturance of a human being in utero. Nelson takes a different route to the conclusion that HETr is wrong in arguing that it violates the proper bodily relationship between persons.

Nelson does not oppose all embryo transfer. He holds that for a biological mother to accept into her womb her own biological child in his or her embryonic stage of development does not seem intrinsically wrong. So, on his view, it is not the transferring of an embryo into a uterus that makes the action wrong, but rather something else, namely, the lack of relationship between the embryo and the potential gestational mother.

Drawing on the work of Karol Wojtyla, Richard of St. Victor, and others, Nelson points out that a person is not an isolated monad but exists in actual and potential relationship with other persons who share incommunicability, a kind of uniqueness. "Recall that incommunicability is the premier attribute of persons and refers to that which cannot be shared. An incommunicable being has a certain metaphysical absoluteness and so cannot just instantiate a type."[10] So even though all of us share in human nature and instantiate the kind "human being," there is also something about each one of us that is utterly unique and unrepeatable. Nelson continues, "In general as incommunicability increases, so does relational exclusivity. There are certain relationships that are incommunicable and exclusive as relationships."[11] The spousal relationship is one such kind of exclusive relationship. It is impermissible to "swap" spouses because a person's spouse, unlike the person's car battery, stands in unique relationship to the person. In a similar way, Nelson argues, the relationship between biological mother and biological child involves a "total bodily union" such that it is impermissible for a woman who is not biologically related to an embryo to gestate this embryo. "In pregnancy, the embryo who is 'of' the mother is incorporated 'in' the mother, who gives her body and person totally. As such, pregnancy invokes the incommunicable exclusivity of interpersonal bodily relationships. The rescuer, despite the best of intentions, enters into a bodily relationship with an embryo that is meant only for its mother, who can never be reduced to just the 'genetic' mother."[12]

Although Nelson's conclusion—that HETr is ethically impermissible—may be correct, I do not find his argument for this conclusion persuasive. Pregnancy is not like a spousal relationship in terms of totality and therefore exclusivity. There is nothing whatsoever wrong with a wife carrying more than one child during a pregnancy, but there would be something very wrong with a wife having more than one husband during a marriage. Marriage involves a total gift of self, a comprehensive union, because marriage always involves a free voluntary choice to create a marital union on the part of the husband and on the part of the wife at their wedding. By contrast, pregnancy does not involve a total gift of self because sometimes a mother does not consent to being pregnant (e.g., unwanted pregnancies) and the human embryo obviously never consents to conception and implantation.

Moreover, it is unclear why Nelson's argument would not apply equally well to breast-feeding a baby that is not one's own biological child. If HETr violates the relatedness of persons, would nursing a child (an activity of great intimacy and connection) also be improper? If not, why not? Adoptive parents raise their nonbiological children from infancy to adulthood (an activity of great intimacy and connection), yet clearly this is permissible. It is unclear why the bonds of embodied persons exclude the permissibility of HETr but allow nursing and postbirth adoption. Nelson may be correct that HETr is ethically wrong, but the arguments he offers do not justify his conclusion.

Ten

Do Children Contribute to the Flourishing of Their Parents?

IS HUMAN PROCREATION A GOOD? OR IS BARRENNESS A BLESSING? Genesis tells the first couple to be fruitful and multiply (Gen. 1:28). But advocates for Zero Population Growth hold that we ought to have two or fewer children. Are children a blessing for marriage? Or do couples need children like hummingbirds need laptops? Is having children a good, bad, or indifferent sort of action? The thesis of this chapter is that procreation is a good, indeed a great good. I argue for this proposition from the idea of personal vocation to love and its connection to suffering, from Platonic understandings of eros, from Aristotelian conceptions of friendship, and from Jesus's teachings on salvation.

THE VOCATION TO LOVE AND THE WILLINGNESS TO SUFFER

God's plan, in one sense, is the same for all of us. The universal vocation of every human being from Adam and Eve to the most recently procreated human being is the shared call to know, to love, and to serve God and other people. In fulfilling this vocation, we find happiness.

In a second sense, God's plan involves different states in life. The vocation as a state in life varies from person to person. Some are called to know, love, and serve God and other people as priests or as religious sisters or brothers. Some are called to know, love, and serve as husband and wife. Marriage is a true vocation. Some are called to know, love, and serve as single people, and this is their true vocation.

Finally, there is a third sense of vocation, personal vocation.[1] A particular man may be called to serve as a Jesuit priest teaching philosophy at Boston College. A particular woman may be called to serve as a Carmelite sister taking care of the infirm elderly at Marycrest Manor. And a particular man may be called to marry Jennifer Turner and to be the father of their children. A personal vocation is utterly unique to that particular individual and to no other. Just as Mary alone was called to be the mother of Jesus, and Joseph alone was called to be the husband of Mary, so each of us is called to some task specific to us alone. As St. John Henry Cardinal Newman put it, "I am created to do something or to be something for which no one else is created. . . . God has created me to do Him some definite service; He has committed some work to me which He has not committed to another. I have my mission. . . . Somehow I am necessary for His purposes, as necessary in my place as an Archangel in his. . . . He has not created me for naught. I shall do good, I shall do His work; I shall be an angel of peace, a preacher of truth in my own place."[2]

A personal vocation is to be husband or wife to *this* spouse, to be father or mother to *this* child, to respond to the specific needs, weaknesses, desires, proclivities, and strengths of those whom God has placed in our lives. The universal vocation of every human person is the vocation to love, and this love is to be carried out by each individual in a specific way in his or her unique and personal circumstances. God has made us for love.

God's plan helps us to find an answer to one of the most important questions a person can ask, "What makes for a good life?" We find an interesting convergence of philosophical, theological, and psychological insight on this question. Though they disagreed about many matters, Aristotle (*Nicomachean Ethics*) and Epicurus (*The Art of Happiness*) agreed that without loving friendships no human being could be happy. In the theological realm, Augustine of Hippo (*Homilies on the Gospel of St John*

7.8) summarized the teaching of Jesus for having a blessed life: "Love, and do what you will" (*Dilige, et fac quod vis*).[3] In his *Summa theologiae*, Thomas Aquinas, like countless Christian theologians before and after, linked loving rightly with living happily.[4] Contemporary psychology also reinforces the centrality of love for human flourishing. The lead researcher of the Harvard Study of Human Development George Vaillant said, "Happiness is love, full stop."[5] Likewise, the founder of positive psychology Martin Seligman emphasized loving relationships as the single most important element of his understanding of human flourishing.[6]

But if living a good life cannot be had without loving, Sigmund Freud was also surely right in saying, "We are never so defenseless against suffering as when we love."[7] C. S. Lewis, though a radical critic of Freud, agreed with him about this matter. Lewis wrote,

> To love at all is to be vulnerable. Love anything and your heart will be wrung and possibly broken. If you want to make sure of keeping it intact you must give it to no one, not even an animal. Wrap it carefully round with hobbies and little luxuries; avoid all entanglements. Lock it up safe in the casket or coffin of your selfishness. But in that casket, safe, dark, motionless, airless, it will change. It will not be broken; it will become unbreakable, impenetrable, irredeemable. The alternative to tragedy, or at least to risk of tragedy, is damnation. The only place outside Heaven where you can be perfectly safe from all the dangers and perturbations of love is Hell.[8]

Not only does loving expose a person to suffering, but suffering for someone can augment love. The "IKEA effect" is the psychological finding that people value their IKEA furniture (which they had to toil to construct) more than furniture that did not require assembly.[9] We love what we have worked for, toiled over, and suffered for. If these insights are correct, suffering and enjoying a good human life are not set in zero-sum opposition. Through their connection in love, to live well and to suffer are not mutually exclusive but mutually implicative.

We can perhaps better see the connection between flourishing and suffering by considering the nature of love. In his book *One Body*, Alexander Pruss proposed that love involves willing the good of the other person as other, appreciating the good of the one who is loved, and seeking unity with the one who is loved.[10] Love's first characteristic, then, is to will the good of other persons as other, to desire the good for them for their own sake. Thus love of enemies is a paradigm case of authentic love, for in loving one's enemies there is no reasonable expectation that they will give us something back in return.

The second characteristic of love, according to Pruss, is appreciation. Willing the good of the other as other is not sufficient for the fullness of love. As the founder of L'Arche Jean Vanier wrote, "To love someone is not first of all to do things *for* them, but to reveal to them their beauty and value, to say to them through our attitude: 'You are beautiful. You are important. I trust you. You can trust yourself.' To love someone is to reveal to them their capacities for life, the light that is shining in them."[11]

Love involves appreciation of the reality of what is good about an individual. If we "do good" for others but hold them in contempt as if they were human garbage, we fail to love them. To love people is to choose an intentional focus in appraising them. "Whatever is true, whatever is honorable, whatever is just, whatever is pure, whatever is lovely, whatever is gracious, if there is any excellence and if there is anything worthy of praise, think about these things" (Phil. 4:8). This focus is compatible with, indeed demands, a responsiveness to reality. I am not really loving my mother if I appreciate her as Prince George of England.

Love's appreciation of others is not blindness to their faults, failings, and foibles but is mindful that everyone is more than their faults, failings, and foibles. As Alexander Solzhenitsyn wrote in his *Gulag Archipelago,* "The line separating good and evil passes not through states, nor between classes, nor between political parties either—but right through every human heart—and through all human hearts. This line shifts. Inside us, it oscillates with the years. And even within hearts overwhelmed by evil, one small bridgehead of good is retained."[12] In the natural law tradition, this inherent bridgehead of good is manifested in the first principle of practical reason always operative in each agent, "Good is to be done and pursued and evil avoided."[13] Every human person on earth is a shifting mixture of the good and the bad, in both moral and nonmoral terms. We can choose to focus on what is bad. But to love someone is to choose to focus on what is good.

The third characteristic of love, according to Pruss, is that love seeks unity with the beloved. Erotic love, friendship love, parental love, and other types of love differ, in part, by virtue of the kinds of unity they seek. Erotic lovers desire sexual union. Loving friends desire to share activities together, like walking, chatting, and working. Loving parents desire to raise their children and watch them in their activities. Lovers of God desire to be unified with the Lord in prayer, service, and theology.

If we understand love in this threefold way, and if love is needed for a good human life, then we have reason to hold that the good life for a human being will always involve suffering. First, to will the good for another person often involves a sacrificial cost to the one who so chooses. To care for the sick, to bear wrongs patiently, and to change for the beloved involves sacrifice. All these acts are sacrificial. Even the most virtuous among us surely finds the demands of willing the good for others as personally costly in time and in effort. Moreover, trying to help others also often leads to disappointment. If we help a student with learning disabilities study for the test, frustration abounds even further if the result is the usual F despite our best efforts. To try to help someone is to risk, and often to experience, the failure to actually help someone. In such cases, our time and effort may well have been put to better use, so this adds to a sense of frustration.

Second, the fragility of human goodness in all dimensions makes the one who appreciates the good of the beloved vulnerable to loss and disappointment. The goodness of health fades into decrepitude, intelligence into dementia, and human life ends always in death. Human beauty, of body or soul, does not endure; as the Bard noted, "Every fair from fair sometime declines, / By chance or nature's changing course untrimm'd."[14]

Finally, suffering arises because our unity with others makes us suffer in compassion when they suffer. When we love our friend, we suffer when our friend is sad, sick, or silenced. Since virtually everyone experiences suffering, our unity with those we love leads us to suffer when they suffer. In sum, human flourishing and human suffering are linked by love that seeks at some personal cost to give to the beloved, that appreciates the fragile good of the beloved, and that is unified with the beloved in times of sorrow. If we are to flourish as human beings we need to will the good of others, appreciate the good of others, and seek unity with others. But if we will the good of others, we will often be frustrated at the lack of success in actually bringing about the good. If we appreciate the good of others, we will often suffer when their good is undermined or corrupted over time. And if we seek unity with others, we will have to endure the compassionate sorrow when they (as they surely will) endure suffering of their own.

We find this mutual implication of suffering and flourishing vividly in the lived reality of married love. Even those in happy marriages can appreciate the grain of truth in the joke "First, the engagement ring, then, the wedding ring, and then, the suffering." Willing the good of one's spouse often involves sacrifice, sometimes heroic sacrifice. Married love appreciates the reality of the spouse, but that reality can disappoint. What makes married love distinctive is not so much willing the good or appreciating the other as the kind of unity that is promised in married love.

In a Catholic marriage, the couple is asked whether they have come to enter into marriage freely and without coercion, whether they will love each other until death does them part, and whether they will accept children and bring them up according to the law of Christ and his Church. Unless the couple promises a love that is free, faithful, and fruitful, the couple is not free to marry in the Catholic Church. This unity as husband and wife, for as long as they both shall live, can cause suffering. As J. R. R. Tolkien observed in a letter to his son, "Nearly all marriages, even happy ones, are mistakes: in the sense that almost certainly (in a more perfect world, or even with a little more care in this very imperfect one) both partners might be found more suitable mates. But the real soul-mate is the one you are actually married to."[15] It is important to remember, lest we have an unbalanced assessment, that every alternative to marriage also involves suffering. The single life can be a lonely life without spouse and children to accompany us. Serial monogamy lacks the depth of commitment for the future and the long history of shared joys and struggles. For most people, marriage, despite its difficulties, characteristically leads to greater flourishing in health, in wealth, and in self-reported well-being than remaining single or divorcing.[16]

HOW DO CHILDREN RELATE TO MARITAL FLOURISHING?

Some people view the procreation and education of children as at best one option among many for married couples and at worst a negative drain on the well-being of the couple. A hedonistic philosophy of life regards marriage with suspicion and children with even greater suspicion. Human flourishing, according to this view, involves lots of sex, drugs, drinking, and lack of suffering. This view of life is represented in the Gospel of Luke by the rich man who advises himself, "Rest. Eat. Drink. Be merry" (Luke 12:19). Here contraception is not just an option but an obligation.

Perhaps no one more notoriously embodied this philosophy than *Playboy* magazine founder Hugh Hefner. He celebrated abortion, extramarital sex, contraception, and self-satisfaction. Yet even Hugh Hefner eventually realized that what he was looking for could not be found in sexual escapades with casual partners. At sixty-three, Hefner married and fathered two children in rapid succession. The *New York Times* reported that Hefner said: "'Having this marriage now and these children, seeing toys in the mansion, I get teary-eyed.' Indeed, his eyes fill and he presses his fingers to his mouth punishingly hard. 'I spent so much of my life looking for love in all the wrong places,' he says, wiping his eyes. Though it should sound trite, it doesn't. The weariness in his voice and the weight in his face suggest the toll of decades of grueling work, of nursing the impossible image of himself as the life of every party."[17]

The life of the party is now dead, but we can learn from Hefner's missteps. Despite his love for his children, expressed in the passage above, his decades of habituation in lack of commitment led to his marriage falling apart before a decade was done. The goods of marriage, like all human goods, are fragile. Given the failure of Hugh Hefner's way of pursuing happiness, as seen eventually even by Hefner himself, let's consider a radically different answer to the question, How do children relate to marital flourishing?

Classic Christian belief emphasizes, in accordance with its Jewish roots, the goodness of having children. According to the Second Vatican Council, "Marriage and conjugal love are by their nature ordained toward the begetting and educating of children. Children are really the supreme gift of marriage and contribute very substantially to the welfare of their parents."[18] Children contribute to the flourishing of their parents in three dimensions: by realizing the goal of erotic love, by providing an opportunity for establishing or strengthening a friendship of virtue, and by helping the parents to preserve and strengthen the gift of salvation.[19]

REALIZING EROTIC LOVE

One of the most memorable and influential views of erotic love is proposed in Plato's *Symposium*. In the *Symposium*, the Platonic Aristophanes tells a story about the origins of erotic love. Once, human beings had four arms, four legs, and two faces. We were like conjoined twins joined back to back. We were so powerful, in our original creation, that we rebelled against the gods. Our punishment for this unsuccessful rebellion was to be split in two, in order to weaken us. This punishment both gave us the form we now have (two arms, two legs, one face) and also gave rise to erotic love, the desire to be as united as possible with the beloved.

Modern ways of speaking about love echo the Platonic Aristophanes. In a 1996 film starring Tom Cruise, the character Jerry Maguire says to his beloved, "You complete me." Couples speak of "my better half" and "my other half." When a relationship fails, we "break up." Erotic love might be defined as seeking to be as united as possible with the beloved, especially in a bodily, sexual way.

To be as united as possible involves being united with the beloved in terms of exclusivity as well as permanence. Love songs speak of "you alone" and "forever." When in the madness of erotic love, one feels as if love will last forever and one wishes for this love to last forever. The beloved of erotic love is utterly irreplaceable, a singularity that cannot be replicated. Moreover, erotic love is a love of the whole person, rather than just love of the other as (potential) sexual partner. If the Platonic Aristophanes is right in his conception of erotic love, it makes sense that erotic love prompts couples to vow to be husband and wife in good times and in bad, in sickness and in health, until death do us part. Erotic love is the desire to be together forever.

Procreation is a way of realizing the goals of erotic love, to be together forever, united to this one alone until death. Erotic love aims for unity, and every child is a living and lasting sign of the unity that once existed between the mother and the father. Erotic love seeks exclusivity and eternity. The one love says to the beloved, "you alone" and "forever." Every child unites the mother to the child's father alone, and the father to the child's mother alone.[20] Every child unites mother and father together forever. Normally, the unity is not merely physical, as if it were a mere matter of shared DNA, but emotional and psychological. Loving parents, whatever their differences, share in having goodwill toward, appreciation of, and desired unity with their children. Even after divorce, many couples still share a love for and devotion to their children.

ENHANCING FRIENDSHIP

In *The Seven Principles of Making Marriage Work,* the psychologist John Gottman, working with empirical data arrived at through observing thousands of married couples in his University of Washington "love lab," wrote that the determining factor in whether a wife or husband feels satisfied with the sex, romance, and passion of their relationship is the quality of the couple's friendship.[21] Friendship could be defined in terms of mutual goodwill, shared activity, and shared emotional life. Having children together fosters marital friendship at least insofar as shared children give the parents an extra reason to have goodwill for each other. Divorce is the death of a marriage, the exact opposite of marital friendship. Having children together is associated with a lesser likelihood of divorce. In his book *The Evolution of Desire,* psychologist David Bess made a similar finding: "According to a United Nations study of millions of people in forty-five societies, 39 percent of divorces occur when there are no children, 26 percent when there is only a single child, 19 percent where there are two, and less than 3 percent when there are four or more."[22] If I have children in my marriage, my spouse is not just my wife but also the mother of my children. In virtue of loving the children, I have an extra reason for loving her. When difficulties arise, as they inevitably do, children provide an extra motivation to make things work. Couples who know that their kids will suffer if their marriage falls apart have extra reasons to seek reconciliation.

The activity of raising children, as well as accompanying them as adults, gives the couple a shared emotional life. Mother and father are united in joy at first Holy Communion, graduation from high school, celebration of a wedding, or the birth of a grandchild. Mother and father are united in sorrow at schoolyard bullying, high school hazing, an arrest of a child for drunk driving, or the unemployment of an adult son or daughter. A child inevitably brings to his or her parents times of frustration and desolation and at other times elation and exhilaration. The rollercoaster ride of parenthood can go from panic, rage, and stress to serenity, tranquility, and exaltation and then back again. Whatever their emotional ups and downs, children benefit parents by providing them resources for a shared emotional life, enhancing their friendship. On the supposition that both the mother and father care about the well-being of their shared child (a defeasible presumption but one that characteristically is the case), the parents are united in joy when the child is flourishing, united in sorrow when the child is not, and united in hope when the child's well-being is yet to be determined.

In book 8 of his *Nicomachean Ethics*, Aristotle famously distinguished between friendships of pleasure, utility, and virtue. We love in friends what is pleasurable, useful, or excellent, and so from a focus on these three things different kinds of friendships arise. Children do not aid a friendship of pleasure, that which is based on having fun and hedonistic experiences; friendships of pleasure, however, tend not to last anyway. Children also do not much aid a friendship of utility, since children usually need our help rather than offer it. But a friendship of utility is, by its nature, a second-rate kind of friendship. In a friendship of utility, I don't really care about my friend as much as the benefits that the friend gives to me. But what about a friendship of virtue? In this friendship, friends care about each other not simply because they give one another pleasure or utility but because of the excellence of the other person.

How do we gain virtue? At least for the acquired virtues, we gain an excellent character by repeatedly doing excellent acts. When a couple has a child, that vulnerable baby needs round-the-clock help. In performing caring, gentle, kind, and loving acts for their baby, their toddler, their grade-schooler, their teenager, and their young adult child, parents grow into more caring, gentle, kind, and loving people.[23] Inasmuch as the couple has more children, they have further opportunity for growth in virtue. Virtue grows through virtuous action. The more opportunities one has for virtuous action the more opportunities one has to grow virtuous. If one has only one child, then one has only one opportunity to help one's offspring through the terrible twos, through riding a bike, through learning to read, and so on. But with each additional child, there are additional opportunities to serve.

Of course, having children is neither a necessary nor a sufficient condition for becoming virtuous. Many of the greatest saints of the Christian tradition (St. Francis of Assisi and Mother Teresa spring to mind) had no children. Nevertheless, parents with children imitate in their own modest way the daily and arduous labors of more famous saints who served the vulnerable in their midst. There is Christian virtue in parents caring lovingly for the needs of their own children. Parents who lovingly care for their physically or mentally disabled children exhibit this virtue in heroic ways. Inasmuch as these parents grow in virtue, they establish or strengthen the basis for a friendship of virtue.

HAVING CHILDREN AND HEAVENLY HAPPINESS

Having children helps a couple in their journey toward heaven, I think, in part by providing an opportunity for deepening faith.[24] Faith is a gift that grows when exercised and atrophies, or even dies, when not exercised. Responsible parenthood, by which I mean a prudent generosity in the transmission of human life, can be an act of faith in God's guidance of the Church and God's providential care for each family.[25] St. John Henry Cardinal Newman wrote:

> Let every one who hears me ask himself the question, what stake has *he* in the truth of Christ's promise? How would he be a whit the worse off, supposing (which is impossible), but, supposing it to fail? . . . What have *we* ventured? I really fear, when we come to examine, it will be found that there is nothing we resolve, nothing we do, nothing we do not do, nothing we avoid, nothing we choose, nothing we give up, nothing we pursue, which we should not resolve, and do, and not do, and avoid, and choose, and give up, and pursue, if Christ had not died, and heaven were not promised us.[26]

Those who accept and live the call to responsible parenthood can say that they ventured living in accordance with what they believed God wanted from them. How many people with three, five, seven, or more children would have had only one or two but for their venture of faith? I know I am one.

If a couple follows the Church's teaching, it is likely that the couple will have a larger family than they would have had if they had not followed the Church's teaching. The reason is fairly simple. If a couple is not using contraception but rather is using fertility awareness methods or Natural Family Planning (NFP) to delay births, then in each woman's cycle a decision must be made to abstain from sexual intercourse during the fertile time of the cycle, during which time she is characteristically more interested in having sex. So, at each cycle, the urges of nature prompt a couple to reconsider their decision to postpone having a child. If the couple has a healthy sex drive, the couple has an ongoing incentive for making love rather than periodically abstaining. Of course, many couples forgo entirely using NFP, as well as contraceptive methods, so for them (again assuming normal fertility and sex drive) it is likely that their family size will be greater than the contemporary average.

If a couple has a larger family, they will almost certainly have a larger share of the emotional highs and lows that accompany having any children. At least for good parents, having children adds something radically new to one's life, an unconditional commitment of love to this particular person until death. So each child a couple has reaffirms in a new way the vows made in marriage: to love in good times and in bad, in sickness and in health, until death. Although no explicit vow is made to the child, good parents have an unbreakable commitment to each child that reflects the unconditional commitment of the marriage vow, in its turn a visible sign of the invisible reality of God's irrevocable love for each of us.[27]

When teenage and adult children cause parents great suffering, their parents may be tempted to waver in their duty to love their children unconditionally. For example, it can cause immense pain and sadness to raise a child in the practice of faith only to see the child turn away from the practice of faith. Elie Wiesel's son, Elisha Wiesel, speaks of his Jewish experience on this point:

> There is a chasidic story of the Baal Shem Tov, who was once approached by a chasid, bemoaning how far his son had strayed. The

rebbe's surprising answer: "Love your son more." . . . My father must have heard this story because he lived it. He believed in me even when I did not believe in myself. He believed in me as I set out on a journey that would take me very far from Judaism and from him. And he believed in me even as I shouted at him that I wanted nothing to do with his religion, that I wanted to be an X factor in every equation he and my mother had used to project my life, that I would be an atheist or a Buddhist, anything but what he told me I had to be. My father kept telling me to be a good student, a good son, a good Jew. But he said it more quietly.[28]

After his father's death, the son felt the presence, love, and guidance of his father in ways even more powerful than when his father was alive. Elie Wiesel must have surely been tempted to stop loving his son, but his fidelity—with God's help—paid off in a son who is guided more strongly by his father's wisdom now than when the father was alive.

Christian spouses can help other people to be open to the gift of faith. In their very mode of living, Christian spouses with larger families can provide testimony by forgoing the vacations and other material perks enjoyed by the typical "two income-two child" family. A martyr is a "witness," a public sign to others of the Kingdom. A priest or nun in distinctive religious garb silently prompts a question in those who see them, "What if they are right about the importance of God? They seem awfully committed to it."[29] A large family communicates a similar message to the world. Life is not primarily about enjoying bodily pleasure, increasing riches, or possessing power.

DIVINE COMMANDMENTS

Jesus taught that the greatest commandment is "Thou shalt love the Lord thy God with all thy heart, and with all thy soul, and with all thy mind" (Matt. 22:37). Love and knowledge are connected, inasmuch as we cannot love what we do not know, and the more we know about the goodness of the one we love, the more we can appreciate the one we love. We are helped to heaven by deepening our knowledge of God.

According to Thomas Aquinas, one path to deeper knowledge of God is apophatic theology, the way of remotion by which we remove misunderstandings about God. Apophatic theology proceeds by denial of characteristics to God. We have a less inaccurate understanding of God when we clear away misconceptions about God. Negative theology is a way of denial in which various terms are said not to apply to God. For example, God is not composed of parts. God has no beginning. God is not a body. These statements reflect the way of remotion, negative theology.

All parents come to realize quickly that their parenthood is not like the parenthood of God. God is not impatient. God is not overwhelmed. God is not at a complete loss about what to do. In coming to know who God is not, in coming to see ever more clearly that we are not God, parents come closer to the true God. We parents come to know in an emotional way that we are not God. To have a deep sense of nondivine status is to open oneself up in new ways to relying on God.

Indeed, children teach parents humility. As young children, we know we are not God. Someone else determines when we get out of bed, what we wear, what we eat, and where we go. When we become adults, it is easier to get the feeling that we are the ultimate arbiters of our universe. As adults, we find it easier to fall into the illusion that we are in complete control. We decide when we get out of bed, what we wear, what we eat, and where we go. We might even come to believe that one has "the right to define one's own concept of existence, of meaning, of the universe, and of the mystery of human life."[30]

Children shatter the illusion that we are God. In his book *Existentialism and Human Emotion*, the philosopher Jean-Paul Sartre held that all human beings have the "desire to be God."[31] This desire to be God is thwarted by children. We do not choose their looks, their native intelligence, their athletic ability, their temperament as introverted or extraverted, their slowness or rapidity to react.[32] We cannot, despite efforts to discipline them, make our children as we might like.

We are also *vulnerable* in our children. Even if we are healthy, their sicknesses afflict us. For parents the good of the child is constitutive of their own good, so when this good is undermined the parents are also undermined. The social and educational traumas of children impinge upon parents regardless of the parents' social class or educational achievement.

Children make the parents feel helplessness. When our children suffer, we parents suffer because we are the ones who are supposed to care and protect but we cannot do it. This can open the parents to call on God, whose care and protection can ultimately save even the most hopeless situation.

According to Thomas Aquinas, another path to deeper knowledge of God is analogy, an understanding of how God is not exactly like but nevertheless similar to created things.[33] For example, in understanding something about human intelligence, we can gain some understanding into the cause of human intelligence. Parents are like God in that they cooperate in giving life. Aside from God, parents have the most power over the lives of their young children, determining virtually every aspect of their lives. In experiencing the powerful, unconditional love that parents have for children, parents can come to realize, in some limited sense, something more about the powerful, unconditional love of God for them and for their children. In understanding the fragility of their children, parents can better understand their own fragility and dependence upon God their Heavenly Father. In seeing the weakness, sinfulness, and dependency of their own children, parents can become awakened to their own weakness, sinfulness and dependency. This opens up the possibility of greater reliance on God.

When Jesus was asked by the rich young man about how to get to heaven, our Lord replied, "If you wish to enter into life, keep the commandments" (Matt. 19:17). Jesus specifically mentioned the fourth commandment, "Honor your father and mother" (Matt. 19:19). Having children helps parents to fulfill this commandment.

It is easy to be critical of one's own parents. They fail at this and at that. But when people have children of their own, they realize how very difficult it is to be a good parent. The stresses and strains of raising children tax our patience and our gentleness and can overwhelm our best intentions. When we have children of our own, we realize that despite our great love for our kids, we often fail them. As we realize our own imperfections, it becomes easier to forgive the imperfections of our own parents. If we, despite our great love for our own children, nevertheless still fail on occasion to give our children what they want or need, then maybe the failures of our own parents were not done because of a lack of love. In coming to understand the challenges of parenthood, we can better understand the challenges that our own parents went through with us. This deeper understanding can lead to deeper love for our parents and so a greater ease in honoring them.

Moreover, in having children, we can come to a deeper understanding of what our own parents gave to us. We can appreciate the enormous time, energy, and efforts it takes to raise children. When we have babies, we realize how much our parents did for us as infants. When we have teenagers, we can perhaps better recall the difficulties we gave our parents as teenagers. The suffering of raising children can lead to greater gratitude to our own parents for having suffered for us. When we are grateful to our own parents, it is easier to give them the honor that God commands us to give.

In the Gospel of Matthew, Christ talks about the Final Judgment. In separating those who are entering heaven from those going to hell, Jesus says to those entering heaven, "I was hungry and you gave me food, I was thirsty and you gave me drink, a stranger and you welcomed me, naked and you clothed me, ill and you cared for me" (Matt. 25:35–36). I remember hearing this passage in church as a child and thinking, "Oh no. Everybody is going to go to hell. After all, who does this? Mother Teresa and her sisters in the Missionaries of Charity will be fine, but everyone else is in big trouble."

Only after I had children did I understanding this teaching of Jesus in a new way. After all, every good mother and every good father do these things on a daily basis. The baby is hungry, and good parents give the child something to eat. The child is thirsty, and good mothers and fathers give their child something to drink. Their son or daughter is naked, and they clothe him or her. How many times do parents bring their sick children to the doctor or hold their hand when they have a fever? And every child comes into the family as a stranger, but good parents welcome the child anyway. So perhaps, on the Judgment Day, the good Lord, having watched our daily toils as mothers and fathers, will say to us, "Come, you who are blessed by my Father. Inherit the kingdom prepared for you from the foundation of the world" (Matt. 25:34).[34]

For good reasons then did the Second Vatican Council echo classic Christian teaching, "Marriage and conjugal love are by their nature ordained toward the begetting and educating of children. Children are really the supreme gift of marriage and contribute very substantially to the welfare of their parents." The Church's message is that having children helps their parents, and these reflections are an attempt to consider various ways in which children help their parents. Specifically, I suggested that having children is one way of realizing the universal call from God to every individual to love. This love, of its very nature, leads to suffering and sacrifice. Children are a gift to marriage and help their parents by (1) realizing the goals of erotic love, (2) providing opportunities for a friendship of virtue, and (3) helping their parents to get to heaven.

Eleven

Is "Death with Dignity" a Dangerous Euphemism?

AS DEBATES ABOUT THE LEGALIZATION OF EUTHANASIA AND PHYSICIAN assisted suicide continue, it may be helpful to examine the terms of the debate more closely. Advocates of physician-assisted suicide and euthanasia sometimes speak of "death with dignity" and the "right to die with dignity." In a certain sense, no one's right to die can ever be jeopardized, for everyone's death is a certainty that no law, no political institution, and no culture can prevent. The "right" to die, in that sense, has no greater need of legal and ethical defense than the right to be subject to gravity. What is at issue is not a right to die, but a right to kill, the legal or moral right to intentionally end someone's life. Not dying (considered as something that inevitably happens) but euthanasia (considered as killing someone putatively for their own good) is the issue. We mean by *euthanasia* or *mercy killing* the intentional killing of a human being, either as a means to an end other than ensuring the death of said person or as an end in itself, undertaken with the motivation of (supposedly) benefiting the one who is killed. The choice to kill may be carried out as either active euthanasia,

119

an intentional *act* such as injecting someone with poison, or passive euthanasia, an intentional *omission* aimed at producing death; for example, withholding the nutrition and hydration necessary for survival. Some forms of intentionally killing the sick, disabled, or suffering are not undertaken for the sake of the sick, disabled, or suffering. These killings are undertaken to help other people, such as those who are tired of caring for the needy, those who wish to save money that would otherwise be spent on their care, or those who look to obtain organs for transplantation. Properly speaking, these cases are not of euthanasia, for in these cases one person is killed for the sake of benefiting another person or other people. We will confine our discussion to euthanasia in the sense of intentional killing undertaken for the sake of the one killed, rather than the intentional killing of one person in the hopes of aiding others.

The right to intentionally kill an individual is sometimes justified by invoking "dignity." Like other words and concepts central to ethical discourse, such as *rights* and *autonomy*, *dignity* is used in a variety of senses. In its root etymology, *dignity* is connected to worth and value. In its contemporary usage, as suggested in chapter 2, we can distinguish various senses of the term, including (i) dignity as flourishing, (ii) dignity as attributed, (iii) dignity as intrinsic worth, and (iv) dignity as equivalent to or at least expressing autonomy.[1] We argue that none of these four senses of dignity justify intentional killing.

Dignity as flourishing is a life lived enjoying basic human goods. A flourishing human life includes acting in ways that are upright, virtuous, and reasonable. So the person who habitually acts with personal integrity has dignity as flourishing in that respect. Daniel Sulmasy puts it as follows: "Thus, dignity is sometimes used to refer to a state of virtue—a state of affairs in which a human being habitually acts in ways that express the intrinsic value of the human. We say, for instance, that so-and-so faced a particularly trying situation with dignity. This use of the word is not purely attributed, since it depends upon some objective conception of human excellence. Nonetheless, the value to which this use of the word refers is not intrinsic, since it depends upon a prior understanding of the intrinsic value of the human."[2]

Dignity as flourishing need not be limited simply to flourishing brought about by reasonable choices. Any human being enjoying basic human goods such as knowledge, friendship, life, and health may be said to enjoy dignity as flourishing with respect to those goods. So a human being suffering from cancer may lack dignity as flourishing inasmuch as her health is failing but enjoy dignity as flourishing in another respect inasmuch as she faces her declining health with equanimity and courageous resolve.

Dignity as attributed can be defined as worth, honor, and respect bestowed upon an individual by the community or by individual choice. As Sulmasy puts it: "By attributed dignity, I mean that worth or value that human beings confer upon others by acts of attribution. The act of conferring this worth or value may be accomplished individually or communally, but it always involves a choice. Attributed dignity is, in a sense, created. It constitutes a conventional form of value. Thus, we attribute worth or value to those we consider to be dignitaries, those we admire, those who carry themselves in a particular way, or those who have certain talents, skills, or powers. We can even attribute worth or value to ourselves using this word."[3]

The president of the United States getting a twenty-one-gun salute, the scholar getting hooded *honoris causa*, and the Olympic champion accepting the gold medal enjoy attributed dignity. The contrary of attributing dignity is dishonoring, shaming, or even torturing particular people because they are viewed as deserving such treatment.

By contrast, intrinsic dignity depends, not on human choice but rather on the inherent nature of the individual in question. Intrinsic dignity follows from the nature of the individual and remains as long as the individual continues to exist. Sulmasy describes it as "that worth or value that people have simply because they are human, not by virtue of any social standing, ability to evoke admiration, or any particular set of talents, skills, or powers. Intrinsic dignity is the value that human beings have simply by virtue of the fact that they are human beings. Thus we say that racism is an offense against human dignity. Used this way, dignity designates a value not conferred or created by human choices, individual or collective, but is prior to human attribution."[4]

We might also call this endowed dignity because it is linked to the nature of the individual and is not achieved by the individual or given to the individual by others. We have endowed dignity or intrinsic dignity in virtue of our humanity, in virtue of our rational nature.

Finally, dignity may be understood as reducible to autonomy. Individuals have this dignity if and only if they have the capacity to choose autonomously. To respect someone's dignity is nothing more than to respect someone's autonomy. As Ruth Macklin argues: "'Dignity' seems to have no meaning beyond what is implied by the principle of medical ethics, respect for persons: the need to obtain voluntary, informed consent; the requirement to protect confidentiality; and the need to avoid discrimination and abusive practices. . . . Why, then, do so many articles and reports appeal to human dignity, as if it means something over and above respect for persons or for their autonomy? . . . Although the aetiology may remain a mystery, the diagnosis is clear. Dignity is a useless concept in medical ethics and can be eliminated without any loss of content."[5]

On Macklin's view, dignity does not do any important work in medical ethics beyond respect for persons. This claim that dignity is a useless concept has been criticized and defended elsewhere,[6] but we do not need to adjudicate that dispute for our purposes. One way, though arguably not the only way, to understand dignity is as a respect for the autonomy of persons. How then do these four senses of dignity relate to forms of mercy killing?

EUTHANASIA AND DIGNITY AS FLOURISHING

Dignity as flourishing involves moral well-being as well as nonmoral well-being. To flourish is to enjoy basic human goods. Human flourishing in its various dimensions presupposes and necessarily involves the human being's continued existence. No individual can have a flourishing life unless that individual is alive. To flourish or fail to flourish qualifies the life. One cannot have a low or a high quality of life without being alive.

But perhaps dignity as flourishing can be used as a justification for euthanasia in the following way. Once flourishing falls beneath a certain threshold, a human being benefits from being killed. We might debate about what exactly that threshold is, and whether crossing this threshold is sufficient for justifying euthanasia or whether autonomous consent is also necessary for justifying euthanasia. The intuition is that once dignity as flourishing has been irrevocably lost, it is better for the one in question no longer to exist at all.

Does illness, provided it is intense enough, make death beneficial? Imagine a sliding scale of human physical well-being. On one extreme, you find Olympic athletes in the flower of youth and the peak of strength, endurance, speed, and every dimension of healthy functioning. As you slide down the scale, this health functioning diminishes to lower and lower levels until it arrives at the other extreme of the scale: human beings just on the verge of complete and irreversible loss of integrated organic functioning in all respects, namely death. The justification of euthanasia in terms of quality of life depends upon the idea that intentional killing, even if authorized by the one killed, is ethically wrong and legally should be prohibited for the Olympic athlete. It is difficult to see why somewhere along the scale of physical well-being intentionally killing human beings becomes not a harm inflicted upon them but rather a benefit to them. How can moving an individual further down the "scale" of physical dysfunction be a benefit to the individual? The further down the scale the individual goes, the worse off an individual is in terms of physical well-being. To kill an individual is to completely destroy the physical well-being of the individual. Killing an individual can never be a benefit to an individual. Benefits make an individual in some respects better off than the individual was prior to receiving the benefit. Intentional killing, by contrast, makes the individual killed not better off but rather nonexistent.

EUTHANASIA AND DIGNITY AS ATTRIBUTED

At first glance, dignity as attributed has little to do with euthanasia. No one views mercy killing as an honor bestowed because of outstanding achievement in service of the public good. Nor is the justification for mercy killing the imposition of a kind of dishonor upon those at the end of life, that they deserve to die because of some bad action that they have done. Euthanasia is not capital punishment.

Dignity as attributed can be used to justify euthanasia in that those who are intentionally killed either no longer have or soon will no longer have any value. If human worth is understood simply as attributed, then it depends upon the judgment and choice of human beings. Just as we can celebrate and honor certain kinds of people, we can denigrate and dishonor other kinds of people. We may, therefore, judge that a certain class of people, for instance those in the last six months of life or those who are enduring grave physical or mental suffering, do not have lives worth living. If certain kinds of human beings, such as those suffering or unconscious at the end of life, have no value, there is no disvalue in killing them, aside perhaps from circumstantial considerations.

Is it true that such human beings have no value? Consider a woman in a hospital in a persistent vegetative state who will soon be dying. Just after midnight, a janitor enters her room and has sexual intercourse with her. Everyone recognizes that this woman would be wronged and her basic rights violated, since it is always wrong to have sexual intercourse with someone without her consent (i.e., to rape someone). But this intuition presupposes that she still has basic rights, that she is still someone who can be morally wronged. In other words, she still has value as a moral subject, despite her grave disability and imminent death.

Dignity as attribution can justify euthanasia only if we assume that human beings do not have intrinsic dignity. We might fail to value something that is in fact quite valuable, such as mistakenly thinking a painting is a knockoff when it is an actual work by Rembrandt. So too, if we classify the gravely disabled as not having value and worth, if we deny them dignity of attribution in a basic sense, we may be making a serious mistake. So the case for euthanasia based on dignity of attribution depends upon a denial of intrinsic dignity to some class of human individuals. For if human beings have intrinsic dignity, there is no human condition for which a basic dignity of attribution is not the proper response. Not every professor deserves an honorary doctorate; but if dignity is intrinsic, every person deserves to be respected, even if the individual in question is suffering, at the end of life, or seriously disabled mentally and physically.

Of course, the suffering person may view herself as lacking any dignity. She may think that she currently is or will soon be worthless and therefore that death is preferable to continuing to exist in her worthless condition. But it is certainly possible that an individual's self-evaluation is mistaken. The anorexic believes she is too fat and may seek help in losing weight. The severely depressed person may think that not only his life but the lives of all human beings lack any meaning, purpose, or significance. If human beings have intrinsic value, then an individual human being may be mistaken in denying his or her own worth.

Another way dignity as attributed may be used to justify euthanasia is by appeal to respect for choices. We acknowledge and realize the dignity of another as attributed by various means such as by providing honors to them, by giving them words of praise, and by granting them social status. Dignity is also attributed when we recognize, accept, and respect the choices of others. In so doing, we treat another person, specifically the person as the source of free and autonomous choice, as having value. So, in cases of voluntary euthanasia as well as physician-assisted suicide, when choices to die are made autonomously, dignity as attributed leads to an acceptance of such decisions as a way of recognizing and reaffirming the worth of the agent as freely choosing his or her own way of dying. To respect other people, we must also respect their own autonomous choices, including their choice to die in the way that they choose.

Though dignity as attributed might be invoked to justify euthanasia or physician-assisted suicide, this justification is problematic. We should recognize and attribute dignity to others in ways that are fitting and responsible. But attributed dignity does not require accepting and respecting all the choices of others, no matter what these choices may be. An autonomous choice can also be selfish, stupid, self-contradictory, irrational, and immoral. We can and should always respect the person who is choosing, but we cannot and should not respect every choice that is made. The choice of the segregationist to exclude African Americans from full legal protection and the choice of the advocate of equality to include all human beings in full legal protection cannot consistently both be respected.

In the case of euthanasia, the full legal protection of all human beings is at stake. Laws allowing euthanasia carve out an exception to the equal protection of the lives of all members of the community, legalizing some cases of intentional killing. Legally permitting euthanasia implies that the vast majority of people's lives are worth fully protecting but that a small minority of people's lives (those who are suffering or nearing death) do not merit the same protection and so may be intentionally ended.

Even advocates of euthanasia do not hold that respect for the decisions of others alone requires acceptance of euthanasia. Legalization and/or ethical permissibility is characteristically said to depend upon not just an individual's choice but also other conditions such as intense suffering, lack of mental illness, or an incurable disease. These qualifications limiting euthanasia may arise from a recognition that political conditions would not allow euthanasia at any time or for any reason. But part of the reason such a policy is so politically unpalatable is that important goods, such as protecting the vulnerable, would be jeopardized by such a law.

Another way in which dignity of attribution could be used to justify intentional mercy killing might be seen by way of analogy. A customary way of honoring a tattered national flag in the United States is to burn it. The rationale behind this practice is that it somehow dishonors what the flag represents to allow it to continue to fly when its condition has significantly deteriorated. In like manner, we intentionally kill an individual who is significantly deteriorating as a way of attributing dignity to the individual. We show dignity as attributed to deteriorating human beings at the end of life by no longer allowing them to continue in their deteriorated condition.

But we honor people by giving them something that is good. It is not honoring someone but dishonoring them to intentionally inflict evil upon them. To "honor" people by intentionally destroying their knowledge, their capacity to play, their friendships, or their appreciation of the beautiful is not to honor them at all, but rather to harm them.

So the question about whether we can honor people by killing them depends in part on whether death is something good or evil for a human being. Like knowledge and friendship, to be alive is intrinsically good for a human being. Indeed, to be a human person necessarily involves being alive, for without life only a corpse remains. We are human beings, living organisms of a particular species. If we have intrinsic value, then these living organisms have intrinsic value. If we are intrinsically valuable, our lives (which are nothing other than ourselves as bodily) have intrinsic value. Death destroys the human being, and so does not benefit a human being in any way. Yes, death may also lead to an end of suffering, but that does not mean that death itself is good. Good can come from evil and evil can arise from good, without good being evil or evil being good. If someone is kidnapped and escapes, such a person may experience what positive psychologists call post-traumatic growth. The victim of the kidnapping may emerge more altruistic, patient, and virtuous. But this growth does not mean that kidnapping wasn't really evil.

Critics may respond that body-self dualism provides an alternative to the view that "we are human beings." According to body-self dualism, "we" are not properly speaking rational animals, organisms of a particular species; rather, "we" are our thoughts, beliefs, desires, and self-awareness. On this view, "we" may be intrinsically valuable, but our bodies are just akin to vehicles in which what is truly "us" (our thoughts, beliefs, desires, etc.) is located. "We" are intrinsically valuable persons, but our bodies are merely animal organisms that "we" inhabit (or with which we are in some mysterious way associated).

In *Body-Self Dualism in Contemporary Ethics and Politics*, one of the coauthors (Robert P. George) provides reasons to reject body-self dualism.[7] One consideration against body-self dualism arises from cases of multiple personality disorder. Suppose an individual human being has two independent sets of beliefs, desires, goals, and memories. This one human being is Dr. Jekyll and also Mr. Hyde. Now suppose a psychiatrist cures the multiple personality disorder, eliminating the Mr. Hyde set of memories, beliefs, and desires. Has the psychiatrist done an act of compassionate healing for which she deserves praise? Or should the psychiatrist be blamed for "destroying a person" and be subject to criminal prosecution for murder? If curing multiple personality disorder is praiseworthy rather than deserving of punishment, then "we" as valuable beings are not really constituted by our thoughts, beliefs, and desires rather than by a bodily human being.

Is burning the flag to honor the country analogous to euthanasia? The key difference is that the flag is just a symbol of the United States. It is a sign of the thing that is being honored, not the actual thing itself. If the United States fell on hard times, experiencing economic collapse and political chaos, it would hardly be honoring the country to destroy whatever good it had left.

EUTHANASIA AND DIGNITY AS INTRINSIC WORTH

Sulmasy holds that dignity as intrinsic worth undergirds the other senses of dignity. Immanuel Kant provided the classic case against euthanasia and suicide in the *Grounding for the Metaphysics of Morals*. Kant writes: "[If a person] destroys himself in order to escape from a difficult situation, then he is making use of his person merely as a means so as to maintain a tolerable condition till the end of his life. Man, however, is not a thing and hence is not something to be used merely as a means. He must in all his actions always be regarded as an end in himself. Therefore, I cannot dispose of man in my own person by mutilating, damaging, or killing him."[8]

Human persons have intrinsic dignity unlike things with a price. Mere things may be used, abused, or even destroyed for the sake of some other end. But human beings must always be respected as ends in themselves and may never be used simply as a means, including being killed or maimed for some other end.

On this view, the value of a human being does not depend on whether the individual is experiencing pleasure, or pain, or nothing at all. Human beings have value not because of what they are experiencing but because of who they are. Indeed, we care about what human beings experience precisely because we care about human beings. If human beings themselves lack value, then why should we care about what human beings experience? The slaveholder does not care about the slave and therefore is indifferent to the suffering of the slave.

Kant's insight might be reformulated. Basic human goods provide the ultimate reasons for action. These basic goods—such as knowledge, health, life, and friendship—are intrinsic goods rather than merely instrumental goods, like money, prestige, and power. But to kill a human being in order to attain some other end is to reduce an intrinsic good to the status of a merely instrumental good. To act in this way is to confuse what is merely a means with what is an end in itself. It is to act unreasonably and immorally.

Euthanasia may be undertaken with various goals in mind: to end suffering, to respect a decision, to save money, to escape from a hopeless situation. But whatever motivates the choice to intentionally kill, the person (in his or her bodily existence) is destroyed, is used up as it were in order to attain this other state of affairs.

The view that euthanasia is impermissible does not entail that all treatments that extend life must always be used regardless of circumstances. To say that every human person has intrinsic worth is not to claim that every treatment offered to a human person has intrinsic worth. In fact, some treatments are more burdensome than beneficial. If a particular treatment is painful, costly, and difficult to administer, this treatment may not be worthwhile for a particular patient. If the burdens of a particular treatment are substantial, and the benefits of the treatment not as significant, then the treatment may be refused or discontinued. The proper judgment is not about whether the *person* is worthwhile, but whether the *treatment* is worthwhile.[9]

Is there a gap between affirming the value of all persons and affirming that the lives of all persons are valuable? Could we not claim that all persons are valuable but that the biological lives of a person has value if and only if the person himself or herself values his or her life?

Such questions presuppose a body-self dualism in which the person is one thing but the person's bodily existence is another. Each individual person is intrinsically valuable, but the biological life of a person has only instrumental value. But human persons are not souls trapped in bodies, or functioning cerebral cortexes riding around in bodies as in a vehicle. A human being is a biological organism, and we are human beings.[10] So if we have value intrinsically, then human beings have value intrinsically and these biological organisms have value intrinsically.

EUTHANASIA AND DIGNITY AS AUTONOMY

Let us assume for the sake of argument that the moral import of "dignity" can be reduced to autonomy. Autonomy can be understood in a variety of ways.

For Kant, autonomy is the self-given law of practical reason, which is the same for all rational beings and binds all rational beings in having a duty to act only in accordance with the categorical imperative. Kant views every human being, indeed every rational being, as something "whose existence has in itself an absolute worth, something which is an end in itself."[11] This insight grounds the categorical imperative, which in one formulation obliges all rational beings to "act in such a way that you treat humanity, whether in your own person or in the person of another, always at the same time as an end and never simply as a means."[12] The duty imposed by the categorical imperative binds all rational agents "as the supreme limiting condition of every man's freedom of action."[13]

To destroy an individual having absolute, unconditional worth for the sake of some (indeed, any) further end, even an otherwise legitimate end such as elimination of suffering, is not to act autonomously but rather, in Kant's terms, to act heteronomously, to act against duty, to act unethically.

In a second sense, autonomy is understood to be exercised in any decision made by an individual who gives informed consent. If a patient understands the reality of his or her medical condition, appreciates the certain and/or likely ramifications of a potential choice, and after due reflection decides to execute a choice, then this choice is autonomous. So if dignity is reduced to autonomy, and someone gives properly informed consent to physician-assisted suicide or voluntary euthanasia, then the value of human dignity supports physician-assisted suicide and voluntary euthanasia. In "The Philosophers' Brief," Ronald Dworkin, Thomas Nagel, Robert Nozick, John Rawls, Thomas Scanlon, and Judith Jarvis Thomson offer perhaps the most famous argument for euthanasia based on autonomy: "Most of us see death—whatever we think will follow it—as the final act of life's drama, and we want that last act to reflect our own convictions, those we have tried to live by, not the convictions of others forced on us in our most vulnerable moment."[14] Our choices determine the value of our lives and the circumstances of our deaths. So respect for our human dignity entails a respect for our autonomy, and this leads to respect for the choices of assisted suicide and voluntary euthanasia. On this view, the value of autonomy trumps the value of human life.

A challenge to this view can be raised by considering the ground for ascribing value to autonomous choices. As mentioned, Bird points out, "Every human agent must attribute worth to his purposes . . . [because an agent] regards his purposes as good according to whatever criteria enter into his purposes."[15] If an agent sees his or her goals as worthwhile, implicitly that agent is also affirming some sense of personal worth. The agent is the source of the action. If the action is valuable, the agent must also be valuable. Alan Gewirth puts the point as follows, "They are *his* purposes, and they are worth attaining because *he* is worth sustaining and fulfilling, so that he has what for him is a justified sense of his own worth."[16] The conclusion is that the "generic purposiveness" of rational action as such "underlies the ascription of inherent dignity to all agents" (including oneself).[17] If this reasoning is correct, then intrinsic dignity undergirds dignity as autonomy. Why should we respect autonomy? The *autonomy* of a person matters only if the *person* matters. But if the person matters as an end in itself, as oriented to the goods which are the ultimate reason for action, then autonomy does not justify euthanasia.

Appeals to autonomy to justify euthanasia are often at cross purposes with appeals to eliminating suffering to justify euthanasia. If it benefits a person at the end of life to be killed, why should this benefit be withheld from patients because the patients cannot consent to receive the benefit? Imagine two patients at the end of life. Both experience intolerable pain. One patient has the competence to give informed consent for euthanasia. The other patient not only suffers physical pain but also suffers from mental illness to such a degree that he cannot give informed consent to any medical treatment. If autonomy is necessary to justify euthanasia, the second patient—the worse-off patient—is not eligible for euthanasia.

On the other hand, if consent is not necessary for euthanasia, then the argument from dignity as autonomy is superfluous in the justification for intentional killing at the end of life. Indeed, justifications of euthanasia are often inconsistent in their appeals to autonomy. If there is no ethical difference between intentional killing and removing life support, since removing life support is permitted for the mentally ill and for minors lacking autonomy, then intentional killing of the mentally ill and minors should also be permitted. Of course, critics of euthanasia characteristically argue that there is an ethical difference between intentional killing and removing life support in cases in which the burdens of the treatment are not worth enduring or bearing in view of its comparatively meager benefits. But this difference is characteristically denied by advocates of the choice to kill. So if removing life support and intentional killing are not ethically different, then consistency demands that whoever accepts removing life support for minor children and the mentally ill also accepts intentional killing of incompetent individuals. Thus autonomy does no real work justifying euthanasia.

Perhaps dignity as autonomy is not a necessary condition for justifying mercy killing but is a sufficient condition. If a competent individual deems his or her life no longer worth living, then he or she may licitly receive voluntary euthanasia or a physician's (or other health care worker's) assistance in committing suicide. What makes a human being valuable is that the human being values continuing to exist, and if a human being no longer desires to continue to exist, then this human life no longer has value. It is wrong to kill an individual because that individual values his or her life. And if the individual does not value his or her life, then it is not wrong to kill the individual.

As John Keown points out, the claim that "a person's life has value only if the person values it" is vague, arbitrary, discriminatory, and dualistic.[18] The claim is vague because our desires are by nature vague, shifting, hard to define, sometimes growing in intensity and then shrinking in intensity. How can we all have fundamental equality as persons if our value as persons depends upon the vagaries and shifting foundation of human desires? The claim that we have value because we value our own lives is arbitrary. As John Finnis notes, "Why not pick out other features which characterize human nature in its flourishing—say linguistic articulacy, sense of humour, and/or friendship more deep, transparent, and supple than friendship between man and dog? Why not then call one or other or some set of these the capacity which, while it is enjoyed, makes us people and 'entitles an individual to be considered a person'?"[19] The claim is discriminatory, for if an individual in his or her bodily existence is valuable only if he or she as a matter of subjective psychological fact happens to desire to continue to live, then some people who are depressed, mentally handicapped, severely intoxicated, or brainwashed in order not to value their own lives are excluded from equality in value with others in the human community. Finally, the claim that our value as human beings depends upon our desires is implicitly dualistic, supposing that "we" (beings who can value) exist only when our desires begin to exist, as if our bodies were mere transporters of the reality of merely mental selves.

If autonomy is a sufficient justification for mercy killing, we have no reasoned justification for excluding nonsuffering competent adults (or mature minors) from euthanasia. If competent people consider their own lives not worth living, on what basis should we exclude them from having a "right to die" just because they lack physical suffering or are not in the last stages of a terminal illness? People may consider their lives not worth living for a wide variety of reasons, such as the loss of a significant romantic relationship or frustrated life plans. Now you or I may not agree with such reasoning, but that fact is completely irrelevant at least according to a purely subjective justification of euthanasia based on autonomy.

CONCLUSION

None of the four senses of *dignity* explored in this essay, namely (i) dignity as flourishing, (ii) dignity as attributed, (iii) dignity as intrinsic worth, and (iv) dignity as autonomy, provide a sound justification of euthanasia. "Death with dignity" and the "right to die with dignity" are dangerous euphemisms masking the reality of what is at issue in these cases, which is not precisely death or dying but intentional killing. Such euphemisms obscure the reality that all human persons are equal in fundamental dignity and that this basic value remains undiminished even at the end of life, even in the midst of suffering. The proper ethical response to human problems like suffering is, if possible, to eliminate the problem, not to eliminate the human. The ethically proper legal response is to accord to every person within jurisdiction the fullness and equality of the law's fundamental protection against intentional killing.

Twelve

Should Euthanasia Be Permitted for Children?

RICHARD JOHN NEUHAUS ONCE SAID THAT BIOETHICISTS "GUIDE THE unthinkable on its passage through the debatable on the way to becoming the justifiable until it is finally established as unexceptionable."[1] The essays examined in this chapter seem to vindicate Neuhaus's observation. Advocates of euthanasia and physician-assisted suicide begin push for legalization by promising careful limits and controlled use, but they eventually seek to transcend these limits.

For example, in his article "Child Euthanasia: Should We Just Not Talk about It?," Luc Bovens transforms the unthinkable into the debatable by arguing that if euthanasia is morally permissible for adults it is also morally permissible for minors.[2] If we accept euthanasia in one case, we should also accept it in the other. Bovens considers a number of objections to extending euthanasia to children and finds these arguments deficient.

First, the Argument from Weightiness holds that minors are not permitted to vote or to buy cigarettes or to drink alcohol. A fortiori, if minors may not make these less significant choices, they should not be allowed to make the more significant choice of ending their own lives.

Bovens responds by arguing that various societies do already allow minors to be involved in decision making about whether to remove life support, and these decisions may lead to their own death. As he puts it, "This involvement is justified on grounds of a right to determine what happens in and to one's body, which underlies the 2002 Law on Patient Rights in Belgium and in other legislations."[3] In other words, we already allow minors to kill themselves through acts of omission, so why not also allow lethal choices of commission?

Boven's response presupposes a false equivalency between declining a treatment viewed as burdensome and killing a patient whose life is viewed as burdensome. To decline a burdensome treatment need not be an act of euthanasia by omission. Moreover, it is one thing to involve a minor patient in deliberative *consultation* about medical options, but it is a different thing to give minors the right of final *determination* of medical options. Moreover, his response does not directly answer the objection to child euthanasia: If children may authorize their own deaths, why can children not also drink vodka or shoot heroin? Drinking alcohol or taking drugs involve relatively minor harms or risk of harm when compared with the certain and more serious harm of death.

A second argument that Bovens considers is the Argument from Capability of Discernment. Not everyone can give informed consent, since not everyone is capable of discernment about the relevant factors making up an informed decision. Minor children, like mentally diminished persons, cannot give informed consent for medical procedures, so they cannot give informed consent for euthanasia.

Bovens finds fault with this reasoning: "I propose that what makes a decision authoritative is (1) that the decision is responsive to reasons and (2) that the agent is the author of her decision, that is, she does not relinquish responsibility and defer the decision to others."[4] If a person can be responsive to reasons and self-determining, this agent can make authoritative decisions and therefore can give informed consent. Yes, children may sometimes be, or even often be, more impulsive and emotional than adults in their style of decision making, but these decisions may still be self-determined and reason-responsive.

However, surely informed consent is more than just being responsive to reasons. Children as young as five can understand simple explanations and reasons for doing or not doing human actions. If a very young child is told to clean up her toys so that she can get a treat, she may very well respond to this reason. Children are also notoriously proud of being the author of their own decisions and desirous of making their own decisions, "I want to do it!" Given Bovens's account of what makes for informed consent, children are unjustly denied the other rights and responsibilities that come with being responsible agents, such as voting in national elections, choosing to marry, having sexual intercourse, and dropping out of school. If children can give informed consent for death, surely they may also give informed consent for dropping out of sixth grade. Death is utterly irreversible, but someone can always return to school.

Bovens considers a third objection to euthanasia for children, the Argument from Pressure. Adults, including those who should be acting as guardians, may apply powerful psychological pressure in order to get children to consent to euthanasia. Parents suffer greatly when their child is seriously ill, so parents may seek to relieve their own inner turmoil by pressuring their minor children into euthanasia. To this objection to child euthanasia, Bovens replies: "First, parents typically cling more to the lives of their children than adult children to the lives of their parents. Second, if medical care is socialised then a child's illness is typically less of a financial drain on a parent, whereas the cost of a parent's care facilities chip away from an inheritance. Third, a third party might reason that the elderly have had their fair innings, whereas a child has seen so preciously little of life. For all these reasons, I would expect pressure on the elderly towards euthanasia to be greater than on minors."[5] Supposing that adults may choose euthanasia, despite presumably greater pressure, euthanasia for minors is also permissible since minors will likely face lesser pressure.

Bovens's reply does not cover many cases. Parent-child social dynamics vary widely. In some cases, children boss around parents. In others, parents boss around children. In many cases, Bovens will be mistaken that children face lesser pressure than adults. In addition, the illness of a child may or may not cause greater financial hardship than a parent's illness. The illness of an elderly person may be borne by public expense; the illness of a younger person may not. In many cases, children may face greater pressure than adults.

Bovens treats a fourth objection, the Argument from Sensitivity. Children are more sensitive than adults to pressure. So if equal pressure is applied, children will be more likely to comply than adults, especially children who wish to please what they take to be the desires of their parents. For this reason, children need greater protection than adults.

On Bovens's view, the Argument from Sensitivity also fails. If we suppose that children will receive less pressure than adults, a difference in sensitivity may not be dispositive. Moreover, this greater sensitivity may lead minors to choose not to get euthanized out of care for parents who may be traumatized by a decision for death.[6]

Even if we suppose that children will be subject to less pressure than adults, Bovens fails to recognize that this pressure will have a greater effect on children, who are, in general, more sensitive than adults to pressure. (This presumably is part of the reason that the age of sexual consent is eighteen, since younger people would have much greater difficulty resisting pressure to have sexual intercourse with an older person.) The fact that this sensitivity may lead some children to choose palliative care over euthanasia does nothing to change the fact that sensitivity of other children may lead them to an otherwise unwanted euthanasia. In all other aspects of life, the greater sensitivity of children merits them greater protection. Why not also in the choice to die?

The final objection Bovens considers is the Argument from Sufficient Palliative Care. The sufferings of children may be adequately alleviated by palliative care, so euthanasia is not necessary in order to relieve their suffering. Why kill the patient when you can cure the patient, at least in terms of his or her suffering?

I agree with the response of Bovens on this point, namely that this argument applies to both adults and children so is not an objection unique to the question of euthanasia for minors. However, we can enhance Bovens's response by noting that palliative care for the young involves special technical challenges.[7]

Bovens then makes a point meriting response: "Legalisation of euthanasia will provide the proper incentive structure for its opponents. They will need to make the kind of palliative care that can alleviate the suffering accessible and affordable to minors, lobby the health sector, and educate palliative care providers in hospitals and hospice care."[8] In other words, the legalization of euthanasia provides a powerful incentive for opponents of euthanasia to make sure that better palliative care is available, so as to reduce the numbers of people who choose euthanasia.

All people of goodwill agree that we should alleviate suffering. However, it is the legalization of euthanasia, not its criminalization, that hampers this shared goal. In killing patients rather than relieving pain, the practice of euthanasia detracts from the practice of palliative care. The more euthanasia is chosen, the less incentive there is to advance methods of palliative care. The more euthanasia is chosen, the less practice physicians have in relieving pain. The more euthanasia is chosen, the fewer people choose palliative care. With less demand for good palliative care, there is less financial incentive for developing new methods of alleviating pain. If euthanasia is legalized, patients, families, and doctors will exert less pressure to improve palliative care because death will be seen as another available option. Most disturbingly, legalized euthanasia undermines compassion for those who suffer. Some people will say to themselves or even say out loud, "Even though euthanasia is legal, this person does not choose it. If she is choosing to suffer rather than die, it is her decision to suffer. Why should I help her when she is not even helping herself?" Legalizing euthanasia endangers and undermines those at the end of life, especially those who choose not to kill themselves.

Like Bovens's article, Udo Schuklenk and Suzanne van de Vathorst's "Treatment-Resistant Major Depressive Disorder and Assisted Dying" seeks to expand the scope of those qualified for euthanasia. They write, "Limiting access to assisted dying to people with incurable *physical* illnesses unjustly discriminates against competent people who struggle with *psychiatric* illnesses that render their lives not worth living to them and that motivate them to request assistance in dying."[9] If voluntary euthanasia for adults suffering from physical illness is ethically permissible, voluntary euthanasia is also permissible for adults suffering from mental illness, such as major depressive disorder. Suffering is suffering whether the cause is a physical problem or a mental problem. Persons with mental suffering would seem to have a greater need for euthanasia inasmuch as their suffering will not be ended by a rapidly approaching death (as for those suffering in the final stages of illness) but could continue for the entire length of their natural life. As Schuklenk and van de Vathorst note, "The fact that they are not afflicted with an illness that will end their lives in the short term means that they do not have a 'natural way' out of their continuing suffering. A patient with late-stage cancer who is denied euthanasia may die not the death she requested, but her suffering will end soon. The same cannot be said of a person suffering treatment-resistant major depressive disorder."[10] Hence, mental suffering with no end in sight provides perhaps a greater justification than physical suffering in the last stages of life.

Is pain relief alone a sufficient justification for killing? It is hard to believe that we should relieve pain against the autonomous decision of the one in pain (involuntary euthanasia). So pain relief itself is not sufficient for justifying killing. Moreover, it is questionable whether euthanasia is properly described as "relieving suffering." To be relieved of suffering, a person must be in a position to experience the relief of suffering. But if a person is dead, then the person no longer has any bodily experiences. The dead feel neither pain nor relief of the pain. They feel nothing bodily. Indeed, they no longer exist at all as bodily creatures.

Moreover, the view defended by Schuklenk and van de Vathorst is inherently unstable. They propose including those who endure mental and physical suffering, but they provide no reasoned justification for excluding other competent adults (or mature minors) who want to die. If competent people consider their own lives not worth living, on what basis should we exclude them from having a "right to die" just because they lack physical or mental suffering? People may consider their lives not worth living for a wide variety of reasons, such as the loss of a significant romantic relationship or frustrated life plans. Now you or I may not agree with such reasoning, but that fact is completely irrelevant, at least according to a purely subjective justification of euthanasia.

Earlier in their article, Schuklenk and van de Vathorst invoke both subjective considerations like autonomy and objective considerations like irreversibility of condition and suffering. But at the end of their article, Schuklenk and van de Vathorst offer almost purely subjective criteria for justifiable killing. They write,

> The following are defensible criteria that could guide those considering to regulate assisted suicide:
> • The patients are competent to evaluate their current situation.

- The patients are competent to evaluate their future prospects based on the scientific evidence available at the point in time when they request assistance in dying.
- The patients' decision is voluntary and informed.
- The patients' quality of life is such that they do not consider it worth living, and the likelihood of improvement is exceedingly small or non-existent.
- The patients repeat their requests over a reasonable period of time.[11]

What these criteria omit is noteworthy. Gone is any mention of irreversibility of condition, or intractable suffering, or death approaching. Aside from mentioning that the likelihood of improvement is exceedingly small or nonexistent, autonomy and autonomy alone does all the work. If patients are competent and informed and no longer consider their lives worth living, that is all that is needed to justify killing them. But if informed consent is all that really counts, invocations of suffering and irreversibility are diversions that serve to make euthanasia more politically palatable but serve no real role in justifying killing.

Now, perhaps we might argue that to want to kill oneself or to request death in the absence of mental or physical suffering indicates a lack of competence, a mental illness undermining the ability to give informed consent to anything, let alone killing. But to make this move is to leave the realm of the pure subjectivity and to begin to evaluate which objective reasons do justify killing and which do not. To focus on objective reasons rather than subjective preferences may undermine the possibility of informed consent for anyone to get voluntary euthanasia or assisted suicide. If objective reasons include respect for the basic goods—including human life—then we have grounds for John Keown's objection to suicide (and by extension assisted killing).[12] If objective reasons include respecting all human beings as ends in themselves and never using them simply as a means, we have grounds for Immanuel Kant's "respect for humanity" objection to suicide.[13] If objective reasons include loving self, neighbors, and God, then we have grounds for St. Thomas Aquinas's classic natural law objection to suicide.[14]

What then does informed consent mean? Is it purely subjective? Or must it be objective in some sense to be truly informed? The understanding of the term described by Schuklenk and van de Vathorst is ambiguous: "Legally, competence is understood as 'being able to review and decide about the case at hand.' Patients need to demonstrate a reasonable understanding of what it is that they request, they need to provide a persuasive justification for their request and they have to persuade three doctors independent of each other of this. Suffering from a psychiatric disease such as a depression does not automatically preclude patients from being aware of what they are experiencing and of what their future prospects are."[15]

The criterion of legal competence is entirely minimal, excluding all but the most psychotic of persons. On the other hand, if euthanasia is permitted only if those who request it present a "persuasive justification for their request" that convinces three doctors, then some competent people will be excluded. Why should competent people who consider their lives not worth living be excluded just because they cannot find three doctors who share their judgment? If what is decisive are people's individual choices and views about whether their own lives are worth living in their judgment, why limit this and burden their choices by insisting on three doctors concurring? In any case, such limits could be, in practice, easily evaded by well-publicized public coalitions of Dr. Kevorkian-style physicians.

Opponents of euthanasia have long pointed to the slippery slope from legalized killing for a small class of patients meeting strict guidelines to, eventually, a larger and larger class of persons getting killed. Proponents of euthanasia now push to make this worrisome prospect a reality. With proponents of euthanasia arguing for assistance in dying for minors and depressed people, the unthinkable is now the debatable, but we can hope and work so that it never becomes the legal justifiable, let alone the unexceptionable.[16]

Thirteen

Does Assisted Suicide Harm Those Who Do Not Choose to Die?

PHYSICIAN-ASSISTED SUICIDE AND EUTHANASIA ARE ALIKE IN BEING forms of intentionally killing innocent human persons. As such, both forms of killing create victims in that the human beings who die lose something of great value, their very existence. Those who love those who have been killed also lose something of great value, namely the persons who no longer exist. If all human beings have intrinsic value and dignity, then the intentional killing of any human being is the intentional destruction of someone of inestimable worth.

But these reflections here are not about those who choose to die. This chapter reflects on what physician-assisted suicide and voluntary euthanasia do to those who do not choose to die. What do these forms of intentional killing do to the disabled who are legally eligible for physician-assisted suicide or voluntary euthanasia? How do legalized killing and cultural approval of choices to die influence the healthy, the able-bodied, and the youthful? The thesis of this chapter is that those who do not choose to die in physician-assisted suicide or voluntary euthanasia can also

143

become victims. They can be damaged and burdened, sometimes seriously, by the legalization and the societal approval of intentional killing in the name of mercy. Voluntary euthanasia places at least seven such burdens on those who do not choose to die.

What is the first way physician-assisted suicide burdens people? In his book *The Paradox of Choice: Why More Is Less*, psychologist Barry Schwartz notes that new choices are not always beneficial in terms of happiness but can in fact become burdensome.[1] The introduction of some choices can lead to feelings of anxiety and loneliness, says Schwartz, rather than experiences of empowerment and joy.

Introducing the legal choice of physician-assisted suicide or voluntary euthanasia places a new burden upon those who are already burdened with serious illness. "Should I end my own life?" is a question of crushing existential burden that the legalization of physician-assisted suicide or voluntary euthanasia places on the hearts and minds of all those at the end of life. Whether or not individuals choose aid in dying, numerous individuals now must struggle with the burden of deciding whether to kill themselves. As these people struggle with the pain, the depression, and the difficulties of illness, they now must also struggle with a new challenge. An elderly woman may ask herself, "Why I am suffering all this, when I could end it all?" She thinks also of her children, and how the nursing care that she requires is devouring their inheritance. "Should I kill myself so that my children will have greater financial resources?" She feels guilty for living. She feels guilty for wanting to kill herself. She feels guilt if she tells the doctor she wants aid in dying. She feels guilt if she does not choose death. In the end, the evidence suggests that most people do not choose suicide or voluntary euthanasia, but the legal introduction of this choice makes more difficult and adds to the burdens of people at the end of life.

The choice of legal euthanasia and physician-assisted suicide also introduces a new burden on the families of those eligible for legal aid in dying. Legalized killing can burden the families of the sick and dying in at least two ways. First, once physician-assisted suicide is legalized, some families will experience a conflict of interest in terms of how to relate to the dying person. Consider the following case. A wealthy widower named Henry George Smith is immobile due to a stroke. He is being cared for in Marylane Manor, where he has access to nursing care twenty-four hours a day, at the cost of $10,000 a month. He has already been in Marylane Manor for two years. Henry's children are aware of all these facts. Henry's children also feel the financial pressure of putting their own children through college. Henry's children may feel so burdened by their financial pressure that they also feel a temptation to mention to Grandpa Henry that they "don't feel it is wrong to end your life." Whether or not they actually speak to their father about this, they are burdened with the ever looming choice.

Consider this variation on the case of Henry. Henry's children say nothing to him, but Henry knows their dire financial situation well. He surmises that they could use his money and so receives physician-assisted suicide without in any way consulting them. Learning of Grandpa's reason for killing himself in a suicide note, the family is horrified. Yes, they could use the money, but they much more desired to spend Grandpa's last years together as a family. They are horrified that he mistakenly thought that he would be better off dead and are disgusted with themselves for not making him better aware of how much he was loved. They are horrified now even at the inheritance, which they now consider "blood money."

Rather than being united in concern and care for those at the end of life, families now face the possibility of division and discord. We can easily imagine a situation in which the daughter wants her mom to receive palliative care and die a natural death. The son, however, wants the same mom to have physician-assisted suicide. Middle-aged people already burdened with caring for dying parents and growing children must now shoulder a new challenge. Families will ask themselves questions like the following:

> If we say nothing to Grandma about "aid in dying," will she take our silence as unspoken approval of her killing herself? If we say, "We will respect whatever choice you make," it may lead her to think that we really don't care whether she lives or dies. If we say, "We think it would be best for you and for the family to receive aid in dying," and she doesn't choose physician-assisted suicide, she will resent us and maybe even cut us out of the will. If we say, "We don't want you to get aid in dying, just let nature takes its course," she may think we don't care about her suffering and (knowing Grandma's tendency to be contrary) she may choose to kill herself because of what we said.

The existential challenges and divisions faced by families in removing life support are intensified and radicalized with intentional killing. Only a small minority of those at the end of life depend upon life support, but many more people will be eligible for "aid in dying." Moreover, many people recognize the profound ethical difference (and until recently in all states legal difference) between on the one hand removing life support (leading to a natural death from the underlying disease) and on the other hand intentionally killing someone as an end in itself or as a means to some other goal.

Let us turn now to a second burden, a financial burden. When intentional killing is legalized, insurance companies can exert pressure on vulnerable patients to commit suicide. In Oregon, for example, a cancer patient named Barbara Wagner was turned down for a remedial drug. However, the insurance company indicated that they would pay for her assisted suicide. She told the *Seattle Times*, "I was absolutely hurt that somebody could think that way. They won't pay for me to live but they will pay for me to die."[2] Before legalization of lethal choices, insurance companies could not exert such pressure to commit suicide. For the rich, the burden of paying for palliative care can be easily met. For the poor, however, financial considerations pose a true burden, a cost imposed by not choosing to die. If the choice to die were not legally available, insurance companies would not be in a position to offer this alternative to patients: die at little expense to yourself or continue to live at great expense to yourself. Those who decline the invitation to kill themselves now continue to live with the added burden of knowing they are choosing to incur greater costs to themselves and to their inheritors.

Now let's consider a third burden, to individuals and to society, the undermining of the basic equality of persons. The Declaration of Independence speaks of all human beings as created equal and endowed with certain inalienable rights. (Although some interpreters claim that the founders meant to include only landowning, white men, I believe this interpretation is mistaken.) An inalienable right is one that cannot be given up or waived or given away. For example, your right to liberty is the duty of other people not to enslave you. The right to liberty is inalienable, which means that even if you give consent to become another person's slave, that person still has the duty not to enslave you. Consent does not enable anyone to violate an inalienable right.

Now imagine we write into law that most people have an inalienable right to liberty, but one class of people, namely those whose skin is darker than a particular shade, do not. No one else has the right to sell himself into slavery, but if your skin is darker than this shade or becomes darker, then selling yourself into slavery becomes permissible. Such a norm, it is obvious, divides the human family into two classes of people, those with inalienable rights and those without.

On the one hand, those with lighter skin merit greater protection from slavery. Indeed, they enjoy an absolute protection from slavery that consent cannot change. On the other hand, those with darker skin merit a lesser form of protection from slavery. For this class of people, consent changes the impermissible into the permissible. If the law reflected this division of the races, would the law not reinforce a basic legal inequality of persons? Would not such laws both create and reinforce racial inequalities?

Now, consider the right to life, the duty of all agents not to intentionally kill. If the right to life is inalienable for all people, then all people share a basic equality, morally and legally. However, if the right to life is *inalienable* for one class of people, those who are healthy, and the right to life is *alienable* for another class of people, those who are unhealthy (to whatever arbitrary degree of lack of health is chosen), then all people do not enjoy equal protection from getting intentionally killed. Such a norm, it is obvious, divides the human family into two classes. People with good health merit greater protection from getting killed. Indeed, healthy people have an absolute protection from getting killed that consent cannot change. On the other hand, people who are ill merit a lesser form of protection from getting killed. For this class of people, consent changes what was impermissible into what is permissible, namely intentional killing. If the law reflected this division of the healthy and unhealthy, of the abled bodied and the disabled, would the law not reinforce a basic legal inequality of persons? Would not such laws both create and reinforce inequalities based on health and disability? Disabled lives matter.

Laws forbidding intentional killing of human beings reflect the basic equality in dignity of all human beings. Physician-assisted suicide and euthanasia carve out an exception to the equal protection of the law enjoyed by all people.

The law is a teacher. When the law teaches that some lives matter but other lives do not matter, that some people are "better off dead," that lesson undermines the basic cornerstone of human society.

In fact, human beings in pain have basic worth equal to that of human beings without pain. Human beings in the last months of life have basic worth equal to that of human beings with years to live. And human beings who do not value their own lives have basic worth equal to that of human beings who cherish their own lives.

This lesson of fundamental human equality, a lesson reflected in laws protecting human beings from being intentionally killed, is a lesson that not all cultures and not all people have learned. Most societies in history divide the human family into two classes of people: those who have basic value and those that do not. In every previous case when we have made such division, we have made a horrible mistake: racism, sexism, colonial exploitation, slavery. The law, the culture, and societal mores should speak with one voice about the common humanity of each member of the human family regardless of race, health condition, age, religion, proximity to death, or disability.

A fourth burden falls on those who are eligible for physician-assisted suicide. The dying may internalize their "second-class" legal status. Elisabeth Kübler-Ross described the fourth stage of grief as depression. People who are facing serious illness often already feel "unwanted" and "unimportant." The vast majority of suicide requests are reversed when pain and depression are treated adequately. But even if sick and unwanted people do not kill themselves, "aid in dying" burdens them with another reason to think that they are "unwanted" and only a "burden." After all, why would a society authorize the intentional killing of some class of people, unless this class of people was considered not as valuable as other members of society, not as in need of protection, not as important?

A fifth class of burdens falls on those who do not have a legal right to die. The legalization of marijuana in Colorado for those twenty-one or older was followed by an increased use of marijuana among those under twenty-one. Of course, correlation does not indicate causation, but when an action is made legal, the social stigma of the action is lessened. With suicide, another fact adds to the danger of lesser social stigma. Suicide contagion is the phenomena that self-killing leads to more self-killing. As an article in the *American Behavioral Scientist* stated: "Research continues to demonstrate that vulnerable youth are susceptible to the influence of reports and portrayals of suicide in the mass media. The evidence is stronger for the influence of reports in the news media than in fictional formats. However, several studies have found dramatic effects of televised portrayals that have led to increased rates of suicide and suicide attempts using the same methods displayed in the shows."[3] A society that legally condones suicide can expect a lessening of social stigma for suicide and greater rates of suicide due to contagion.

These social facts influence even those who do not have a legal "right to die." Such persons may think to themselves that they are being denied their "rights." Their actions, though technically not yet legally permitted, are in reality no different from physician-assisted suicide. They may recognize that the legal lines drawn about when a person has a "right to die" are arbitrary. If physician-assisted suicide is legal when a patient has only six months to live, why shouldn't it also be legal for patients with longer to live, since these patients will suffer for a longer time? If there is a "right to die," then why should only those at the very end of life be able to exercise it? If the suffering caused by cancer justifies self-killing, why not the suffering caused by losing the girl of your dreams? After all, if given a choice between having cancer or losing Juliet, we all know what Romeo would choose.

What are we saying to young people, when we legalize assisted suicide? We are telling them that suicide is acceptable, which opens the door for them to conclude that it is choice-worthy. We should not be surprised if suicide rates—of both young and old—increase if legal and moral cultures accept suicide and voluntary euthanasia. The suicide, especially of young people, brings unimaginable pain to those who love them.

A sixth kind of harm that comes to those who do not choose euthanasia concerns palliative care. All people of goodwill agree that we should attempt to relieve the suffering of human persons. Physicians and researchers have increased the effectiveness of palliative care to an amazing degree in recent decades. But if physician-assisted suicide and voluntary euthanasia are legal options, the drive to improve palliative care may be weakened. In general, the more demand that there is for a medical service, the more attention, energy, and development are sought for that service. But the more people at the end of life who choose aid in dying, the less demand there is for palliative care. The more people who choose aid in dying, the less practice physicians have in administering palliative care. The more people choose aid in dying, the less incentive there is for pharmaceutical companies to develop better drugs to treat pain. In these ways, the cultural drive for better palliative care may be weakened by intentional killing at the end of life. Once physician-assisted suicide is a legal option, at least some people will think, "Why should I care about their suffering, when even they don't care about their own suffering enough to end it?" Some people will view those suffering at the end of life, not as noble victims making the best of a difficult situation, but as stubborn and confused dolts who do not choose the easy way out. Why should public monies be spent for palliative care for such people when they can simply choose to end their own lives?

Finally, the last burden falls on those who are killed without consenting to be killed. The moral and legal lines drawn between permissible and impermissible forms of mercy killing cannot sustain the protection of potential victims of nonvoluntary euthanasia. The argument for physician-assisted suicide typically rests on the informed consent of the patient to receive medical treatment from his or her physician. In fact, physician-assisted suicide is not properly described as a "medical treatment" because it does nothing to restore health or proper functioning to a patient. But let's set that difficulty aside for a moment. If physician-assisted suicide is justified because of the autonomy of the patient, why should this autonomy not also justify voluntary euthanasia? In some cases, a patient requests aid in dying but cannot carry out an act of suicide by his or her own hand. Since the patient is too disabled to kill himself or herself, the doctor intentionally kills the patient at the patient's request, for example, by lethal injection. If physician-assisted suicide were permissible but not voluntary euthanasia, we would have the paradoxical situation of the better-off person (who is still able to kill himself) having a right to die and the worse-off person (who is unable to kill himself) lacking the right to die. This is hard to believe. So if physician-assisted suicide is permissible, then voluntary euthanasia is also acceptable.

If these premises are granted, then nonvoluntary euthanasia is also permissible. For in many cases, doctors intervene on a patient without voluntary consent, on the presumption that the intervention is in the best interests of the patient. But the permissibility of physician-assisted suicide and voluntary euthanasia rests on the presumption that killing can be in the best interest of the patient. Indeed, the person who cannot even give informed consent to physician-assisted suicide or voluntary euthanasia is presumably in a more seriously disabled condition, and in greater "need" of aid in dying, than those who can give consent. So if voluntary euthanasia is permissible but not nonvoluntary euthanasia, we have a paradoxical situation. The better-off person (who can consent) has a right to die, and the worse-off person (too sick to consent) lacks the right to die. This is counterintuitive. So the legalization of "aid in dying" cannot logically be limited simply to those who give voluntary consent to "aid in dying." The culture of death instantiated in legal euthanasia extends also to those who do not consent to dying. Legalized killing *with* consent leads to legalized killing *without* consent.

CONCLUSION

A society that legalizes and approves physician-assisted suicide and voluntary euthanasia also produces victims who do not consent. Among these seven burdens is that the sick and disabled will feel that others do not value them any longer. Such persons, already suffering at the end of life, now suffer an additional challenge. The right to die, for them, becomes a duty to die. If they do not act on the pressure placed on them by others, they suffer the guilt of disappointing them. In addition, the legalization of "aid in dying" opens the door to insurance companies putting financial pressure on those at the end of life. Legalization also undermines the fundamental equality of all persons under the law by teaching that some lives are not worth living, some human beings are not worth protecting. Some families will suffer the trauma of a loved one who kills himself or herself in the mistaken supposition that the family would be better off without him or her. A culture that approves suicide can expect more suicide among the young as self-killing loses its stigma. These suicides will devastate many of the families and friends whom they leave behind. Mercy killing also lessens the demand for palliative care and societal sympathy for those suffering at the end of life. Finally, legalized killing cannot be consistently confined to those who consent.

Fourteen

Is Conscientious Objection to Abortion Like Conscientious Objection to Antibiotics?

ONE OF THE MOST PRESSING ISSUES DEBATED IN CONTEMPORARY bioethics is the rights of conscientious objectors in health care. Alberto Giubilini, coauthor of the well-known defense of infanticide titled "After-birth Abortion: Why Should the Baby Live?," has written an article challenging conscientious objection to abortion.[1] In "Objection to Conscience: An Argument against Conscience Exemptions in Healthcare," Giubilini maintains that it is not consistent to allow conscientious objection to some procedures (procuring abortions) but not other procedures (prescribing antibiotics): "Think of a doctor who has a conscientious objection to administering antibiotics because she conscientiously believes that bacteria have significant moral status, and actually a moral status comparable to that of a foetus. I take it that most, perhaps all of us would say that this kind of objection should not be granted."[2]

If no conscience protection should be given to those who object to antibiotics, then there must be some important difference between the antibiotic objector and the abortion objector. Giubilini argues that there is, in fact, no important ethical difference between them. So since we would not allow the antibiotic objector to not prescribe antibiotics, we should also not allow the abortion objector to not perform abortions: "Defenders of conscientious objection *qua conscientious* need to say the no-harm principle constrains the right to object to antibiotics but not the right to object to abortion."[3] However, Giubilini provides no arguments regarding why they must make such an argument.

One way to respond to Giubilini is to say that both the abortion objector and the antibiotic objector may decline to provide the requested procedures: Why not say that a doctor who has a conscientious objection to antibiotics does not need to prescribe antibiotics? This stance would have absolutely no practical consequences for any patients or doctors and removes the inconsistency objection.

Giubilini accepts that health care providers may conscientiously object to some procedures but only if the objection is based on medical principles such as nonmaleficence:

> I have also argued that objections by [health care professionals] are sometimes justified. They are justified—which means that objections should be respected and that good doctors should put them forward—only when the practice to which doctors object violates principles and values of the profession. I have provided two examples of such justified objections, namely objection to providing medical assistance in death penalty and objection to releasing refugees back to refugee camps when this would be detrimental to their health. What justifies the objections in such cases is some substantial value and principle informing the profession, and not values or principles related to the formal notion of conscience such as moral integrity, dignity, or freedom of conscience.[4]

Giubilini's view on this point is inconsistent with his earlier criticism of the antibiotic objector who appeals to the principle of nonmaleficence when declining to kill bacteria. Giubilini should either allow physicians to withhold antibiotics and not participate in the death penalty, since both violate the principle of nonmaleficence, or he should not allow them to refuse either.

Another reply to Giubilini's challenge is that there are significant differences between bacteria and human beings. The Declaration of Independence holds as a self-evident truth that "all men are created equal" and "endowed . . . with certain inalienable rights." It is hardly a self-evident truth that all bacteria are created equal and endowed with inalienable rights. Giubilini seeks to dispel this concern: "One might argue that one value of medicine that could justify opposition to abortion is the special value attributed to human life, which would yield an ethical principle that prescribes to preserve human life whenever possible."[5] Giubilini points out that the medical profession does not require that all human life be preserved regardless of the consequences.

Unfortunately, Giubilini distorts the relevant ethical principle. The claim that human beings have special value and should not be intentionally killed is not the same as the claim that doctors must preserve human life whenever possible. Arguably, the claim that all human beings have equal basic value and should be accorded basic rights is a fundamental principle of Western civilization. Giubilini misconstrues the inviolability of life (innocent human beings deserve protection in law from being intentionally killed) as a form of vitalism (all human lives must always be extended as much as possible regardless of the burdens and benefits of treatment).[6] The claim that no innocent life should be taken is not the claim that everything possible must be done to extend everyone's life in every circumstance.

Giubilini's case for abolishing conscience protections continues: "Doctors who refuse to provide an abortion to a woman who requests it are typically refusing to provide a medical service that is safe, beneficial, and autonomously requested by the woman; therefore, they are acting against the ethical standards of beneficence and respect for patient autonomy which are commonly accepted in contemporary Western medical ethics and medical deontological codes."[7] Is it true that not performing an abortion violates patient autonomy? Does refusing to perform an abortion violate a patient's autonomy simply because the patient requests one? Doctors not only may but must deny some autonomous requests: for example, when a patient wants oxycodone for recreational use.

The beneficence of abortion is also questionable. It never benefits the prenatal human being, and doctors who object to abortion typically do not agree that it is safe for women.[8] Even Giubilini implicitly acknowledges that late-term abortions carry significant physical and psychological risks: "Abortions at an early stage are the best option, for both psychological and physical reasons."[9] Is early abortion safe? Abortions cause an increased rate of ectopic pregnancy, which is a leading cause of death among pregnant women.[10] Even if abortions are safe, beneficial, and autonomously requested, Giubilini's defense of forcing health care workers to perform them makes inconsistent appeals to authority: "In fact, abortion is a procedure that is permitted by many medical associations and that can be performed, as the American Medical Association prescribes, in accordance with good medical practice; it is also commonly taught in medical schools in many countries. How could the institution of medicine condone something like abortion if the prescription to try to save all forms of human life was a core principle of the profession? An absolute prohibition to kill a fetus is not consistent with principles of contemporary medicine and is not itself a principle of contemporary medicine."[11]

Giubilini is correct that the contemporary medical establishment permits abortion. However, these same institutions as well as the law in the United States also permit conscientious objection to abortion:

> Most states have "conscience clauses," which describe a right of refusal for physicians, and in some cases for other providers and for health care organizations such as religious hospitals. Most of these state laws, as well as similar conscience clauses in federal statutes, professional codes of ethics, and institutional policies, were enacted after the passage of *Roe v. Wade* in 1973 to permit physicians to opt out of performing or participating in legalized abortions. Today, most medical students opt out of learning how to perform abortions, as they are permitted to do under the American Medical Association's code of ethics.[12]

So an absolute prohibition of conscientious objection to abortion is neither consistent with nor included among the principles of contemporary medicine. The authorities to which Giubilini appeals to argue that abortion is permissible also allow conscientious objection to abortion. So Giubilini incorrectly claims that "as far as consistency with professional values is concerned, opposition to abortion is no different from opposition to antibiotics on grounds of moral status."[13] No federal statutes, professional codes of ethics, or institutional policies protect antibiotic objectors. No medical students refuse in conscience to learn how to prescribe antibiotics. Moreover, Giubilini's argument inconsistently appeals to contemporary practices. Western medical ethics does not require conscientiously objecting physicians to perform abortions as an expression of beneficence and respect for patient autonomy. Doctors also retain a rightful autonomy, including the freedom not to violate their consciences by performing abortions.

Let us return to the heart of Giubilini's case, that prenatal human beings and bacteria are in relevant ways alike:

> Consider the following description of a patient's condition. Suppose there is a woman who has a parasitic organism in her body—call this organism x. The organism is causing her a lot of distress and is affecting and probably will affect her mental and physical health and her plans in the short and/or in the long term. The woman needs and wants to get rid of x so as to restore her good health. This description fits both the case of a woman asking for abortion and that of a woman with some bacterial infection. In one case x is a foetus, in the other it is a bacterium.[14]

According to this way of thinking, both the antibiotic objector and the abortion objector refuse to eliminate a parasitic organism that is causing distress.

Let us set aside the dehumanizing and degrading rhetoric in which a prenatal human being is called a parasite. To depend on another person for continued existence, as do newborns and also some kinds of conjoined twins, is not to lack human dignity. While it is true that a prenatal human being and a bacterium are both organisms that depend on the body of another, they are different in important, widely recognized ways. Countless medical professionals, such as those specializing in maternal-fetal medicine, dedicate their time and talent to healing and preserving the lives of prenatal human beings. By contrast, there are no neonatal intensive care units for bacteria or ultrasound photos of growing bacteria put on refrigerators, and I have never heard of anyone suffering depression after miscarrying her bacteria. Indeed, in circumstances other than abortion, for example, a car accident in which a pregnant woman is injured, doctors work to save not only the woman but also the prenatal patient. In circumstances other than abortion, the law in the United States protects human beings in utero.[15] For example, the law treats the murder of a pregnant woman as a double homicide. None of this is true of bacteria.

There is another significant difference between prenatal human beings and bacteria. It is a sign not of health but rather of a lack of health when a woman's body cannot successfully sustain a pregnancy. Conversely, it is a sign of health when a woman of reproductive age can become pregnant. A pregnant woman does not suffer from a disease, and the son or daughter in utero is not a parasite working against the well-being of her body. If a woman is healthy, her body is working, successfully functioning to sustain her progeny. It is abortion that introduces a pathology by interrupting the healthy functioning of the woman's body in sustaining the pregnancy. In contrast, by killing bacteria, antibiotics restore healthy functioning and aid the body in doing what it often does unaided: destroy bacteria.

Is objection to abortion more reasonable than objection to antibiotics? Giubilini thinks not: "Using coherence with empirical data as criterion for reasonableness would yield the same response, since we have no evidence at all in support of claims about souls in foetuses. Unless we can explain what makes certain religious views based on unproven metaphysical assumptions more reasonable, i.e. more coherent with empirical data, than other religious or metaphysical views to which we are simply less accustomed, we don't have a principle we can use to discriminate between different cases of conscientious objection."[16]

Giubilini introduces two different standards of reasonableness. To be supported by empirical data is not the same as to be coherent with it, that is, not contradictory to it. Each claim is problematic but for different reasons.

To claim that a view is unreasonable if not supported by empirical data is self-defeating, because this account of reasonableness is not supported by empirical data. No experiment establishes the philosophical belief that reasonableness means being supported by experiments. No scientific study proves that scientific reasoning is the only legitimate form of inference. "Science alone provides the truth" is a statement that science alone does not establish as true. So even if it were true that there is no scientific evidence for the soul of a fetus—or a newborn or a teenager—this lack of empirical evidence does not make the view unreasonable.

A second and very different understanding of reasonableness appealed to by Giubilini is coherency with empirical data. However, he does not cite a single study or finding of the empirical sciences that conflicts with the belief that an individual human being has a soul. The empirical data about fetal development are entirely compatible with belief in a soul. No known biological, psychological, or physiological fact contradicts this belief. If the soul is immaterial, it cannot be directly studied by empirical science (though the empirical effects flowing from the soul such as self-movement could be studied empirically). If we define the soul as immaterial, we could argue—philosophically not scientifically—that souls do not exist by presupposing a philosophical premise that only material things exist or that nothing beyond nature exists. It may be that Giubilini presupposes materialism and naturalism to be true, but he surely must know that many reasonable people deny these philosophies, as Alvin Plantinga makes clear in his book *Where the Conflict Really Lies: Science, Religion, and Naturalism.*[17]

Finally, even if Giubilini is right that belief in souls is unreasonable, the soul does not need to be invoked and typically is not invoked to justify opposition to abortion. To give one example, Don Marquis, an atheist, defends the future-like-ours argument against abortion, which relies on the premise that killing you or me is wrong because it deprives us of our valuable future.[18] If someone kills us now, we are deprived of the friendships and family times, meals and movies we would have enjoyed for the rest of our lives. If allowed to live, the human fetus and the human newborn also have a future like ours, so killing them is wrong for the same reason killing you or me is wrong. This argument does not invoke the soul, and it does not apply to bacteria, which do not have a future like ours. Indeed, virtually no contemporary philosophical critique of abortion presupposes belief in the soul,[19] so it is hard to see why Giubilini makes critique of belief in souls so central to his case for taking away health care workers' right to not perform abortions. In doing so, Giubilini attacks a straw man.

Finally, it is worth recalling that Giubilini holds that abortion and infanticide are ethically similar insofar as neither the prenatal human being nor the newborn human being is a person with a right to life. In his view, "The same reasons which justify abortion should also justify the killing of the potential person when it is at the stage of a newborn."[20] So if his analysis of conscience protections is correct, doctors who conscientiously oppose infanticide should nevertheless be forced to kill healthy newborn infants. If the reasons justifying abortion are also compelling for infanticide and if conscience protections do not exempt doctors from performing abortions, then conscience protections do not exempt doctors from performing infanticides.

Is it reasonable to force an unwilling doctor who conscientiously rejects infanticide to kill a healthy baby after she is born? If it is not reasonable, then we should reject Giubilini's views on conscience, his views on abortion and infanticide, or his views on both.

Fifteen

Do Medical Conscientious Objectors Differ from Military Conscientious Objectors?

INFLUENTIAL ARTICLES IN PRESTIGIOUS JOURNALS CAN SHAPE OR EVEN transform a discussion. In their *New England Journal of Medicine* article "Physicians, Not Conscripts: Conscientious Objection in Health Care," R. Y. Stahl and E. J. Emanuel argue that health care professionals who are unwilling to perform medical interventions to which they conscientiously object, such as abortion, should be forced to leave the practice of medicine.[1] They write, "Health care professionals who are unwilling to accept these limits have two choices: select an area of medicine, such as radiology, that will not put them in situations that conflict with their personal morality or, if there is no such area, leave the profession."[2] What are their grounds for taking away rights of conscientious objection in health care?

Stahl and Emmanuel argue that appeal to conscientious objection in the military has justified and legitimated conscientious objection in health care. Their strategy is to show disanalogies between military service and health care so as to delegitimize conscientious objection in medical practice. Conscientious objection in health care differs from the conscientious objection in the military context in five important ways. Stahl and Emmanuel write: "First, it objects to professional practices, not state-mandated conscription; second, it occurs within the context of a freely chosen profession; third, it allows selective objection to professionally accepted interventions; fourth, it accepts objection without external scrutiny; and fifth, it shields the objector from all repercussions and costs."[3] On their view, these five differences between conscientious objectors in the military and in medicine undermine the case for allowing health care professionals the right to decline to perform requested interventions.

The case of US Army corporal Desmond T. Doss calls into question much of Stahl and Emmanuel's argument. The movie *Hacksaw Ridge* tells the true story of Corporal Doss, who volunteered to serve in the field of combat during World War II. Because of his personal beliefs as a Seventh-Day Adventist, Doss refused to kill or even carry a weapon into combat. Doss was assigned to serve as a medic and received the honor of a Bronze Star for his heroic service on Guam and in the Philippines. In the Battle of Okinawa, Doss remained unarmed among the enemy and single-handedly lowered seventy-five wounded servicemen from Hacksaw Ridge to safety. Doss became the only conscientious objector during World War II to receive the military's highest award for valor, the Medal of Honor.

Cases of conscientious objection such as Doss's undermine several of the key claims of Stahl and Emmanuel's argument. First, Doss objected to normal professional military practices (e.g., carrying weapons and killing enemy soldiers). Second, Doss freely chose military service. Third, Doss selectively objected to professionally accepted interventions by refusing to kill the enemy while still performing all other duties compatible with his religious beliefs.

Stahl and Emmanuel suggest a fourth difference between military and medical conscientious objection. Military conscientious objectors are scrutinized about the sincerity of their beliefs, but medical conscientious objectors are not scrutinized about the sincerity of their beliefs. This difference makes sense. In the case of military service, someone may lie about opposition to killing because of fear of risking life and limb, rather than from sincere ethical belief. In the case of medical service, the motivation to lie in order to avoid the risk of personal injury or death in battle is not present. There is a very obvious ulterior motive for lying in the case of military service but not in the case of medical service. Therefore, scrutinizing a claim of conscientious objection makes sense in the military context but not in the medical context.

And what of the fifth and final difference, that in medical contexts the objector is shielded from all repercussions and costs, but in the military context the objector is not shielded from all repercussions and costs? If the movie *Hacksaw Ridge* is to be believed, Doss certainly was not shielded from all repercussions and costs. In addition to received harassment and even physical assault for his conscientious objection, Doss received officially imposed penalties. It is questionable whether such treatment of conscientious objectors is justified in the military context. If such treatment is not justified, then the precedent of such treatment cannot serve as a justification for extending such costs into the medical context.

In any case, is it true that those in the health care profession who conscientiously refuse to provide abortion are shielded from all repercussions and costs? No, conscientious objectors incur financial opportunity costs because they do not receive the payment they would have received for performing abortion, and they must forgo certain job opportunities such as working in Planned Parenthood abortion clinics. Moreover, to the degree that abortion is a medically accepted practice, conscientious objectors risk social stigmatization in the profession. Conscientious objectors may also undergo termination of professional relationships with patients, colleagues, and hospitals. As things now stand, it is not accurate to claim that conscientious objectors in medicine do not suffer for their beliefs and actions.

Stahl and Emmanuel suggest that "health care conscience clauses are one-sided, protecting only those who refuse to treat patients, not those who conscience compels them to provide medically accepted but politically contested care."[4] Is this claim true?

In fact, the existing conscience protections for health care professionals serve not just conscientious objectors but the whole community. First, conscience protections serve many patients who seek out health care providers with whom they share ethical values and religious beliefs. Many patients feel more comfortable sharing private and intimate details of their lives (as can be so important in health care) with like-minded health care professionals. Such trusting relationships promote the well-being of patients.

Second, conscience clauses protect the diversity of the health care profession, a concern widely shared by people inside as well as outside the profession. Women, Latinos, and African Americans have, on average, higher degrees of religiosity than white men. Religious belief and practice often, but of course not always, motivate conscientious objection. If we want a medical profession that reflects the religious and ethnic diversity of American society, then we should protect the right of conscience of health care workers. Taking away health care protections will in effect make the medical profession more white, male, and atheistic.

Moreover, health care conscience protections for individuals and institutions aid everyone, but especially the disadvantaged, by preventing higher health care costs. For example, "615 Catholic hospitals account for 12.5% of community hospitals in the United States, and over 15.5% of all U.S. hospital admissions."[5] Countless other individual physicians, nurses, and health care professionals share the Catholic opposition to abortion. If these individuals and institutions are forced to provide abortions or stop providing health care, then many of these individuals and institutions will (as Stahl and Emmanuel seem to desire) be forced out of the health care profession. At a time when health care demand is increasing, the Stahl-Emmanuel proposal would bring about decreasing health care supply. Higher health care costs and more difficulty in obtaining health care harms everyone, including women wanting abortions. The woman seeking an abortion may find that her chosen doctor is not only not providing abortion but also not providing cancer screenings, oral antibiotics, or asthma inhalers.

Stahl and Emanuel claim that the conscience protections don't "protect" those who consciences impel them to provide requested interventions. The authors may have in mind doctors working at Catholic hospitals who want to procure abortions. But the case of doctors in Catholic hospitals who want to perform abortions and that of doctors who do not want to perform abortions are in an important way not analogous. There is a radical difference between not practicing medicine in a particular hospital and not practicing medicine at all.

Stahl and Emmanuel remind their readers, "All their professional health care societies accept the same professional role morality: patients' well-being is their primary interest."[6] The coauthors note that the

American Medical Association does insist that the "physician's ethical responsibility [is] to place patients' welfare above the physician's own self-interests."[7] But obviously the primacy of the patient is not an exceptionless principle, as if every patient's interest trumps every physician's interest in every case. It is in the interest of patients to have medical care provided cost-free, but doctors do not have an obligation to work only on a voluntary basis. It is in the interest of patients to avoid the hassle and expense of visiting the doctor's office, but physicians do not have an obligation to provide house calls. It is in the interest of patients to have the doctor see them whenever patients desire to be seen, but physicians do not have an obligation to always be available upon request.

So how important is the interest of a doctor in not providing abortions? Well, conscientious objectors view not providing abortions as more important than not making house calls, not charging patients for medical services, and not providing medical advice off hours in social situations. House calls, free medical treatment, and mid-dinner consults are not matters of conscience for most people. They are not intrinsically evil. So if we allow physicians to let their interest in a family dinner trump a patient's interest in medical advice, we should not force a doctor who thinks an abortion is intentionally killing an innocent human being to perform abortions.

If there is an actual or perceived conflict between doctor and patient, who determines in a particular case whose interests should prevail? Stahl and Emmanuel answer that "the profession, rather than the individual practitioner, elucidates the interpretation and limits of the primary interest (AMA Code of Medical Ethics Opinion 1.1.1)."[8] It is odd that Stahl and Emmanuel should appeal to professional standards to adjudicate conflicts between a patient's interest in getting an abortion from a particular provider and a health care professional's interest in not providing an abortion, since this standard contradicts the view advocated by Stahl and Emmanuel. If the profession elucidates the interpretation and limits of the patient's interest, then health care professionals should be permitted to decline to perform abortions, since the American Medical Association allows health care professionals to decline to perform abortions.

Stahl and Emmanuel go on to argue that the American Medical Association is inconsistent in asserting "fidelity to patients and respect for patient self-determination" as well as protection for health care professionals who object in conscience to being forced to perform abortions. On the one hand, the American Medical Association urges doctors to place patient well-being above self-interest and forbids doctors from rejecting patients on the basis of "race, gender, sexual orientation, or gender identity, or other personal or social characteristics that are not clinically relevant to the individuals' care" (Opinion 1.1.2).[9] On the other hand, according to Stahl and Emmanuel, the American Medical Association contradicts itself: "Conversely, it [the AMA] permits physicians to refuse to treat patients who are seeking care that is 'incompatible with the physician's deeply held personal, religious, or moral beliefs' (Opinion 1.1.2[a])."[10] Is there really a contradiction?

In fact, Stahl and Emmanuel create an apparent contradiction in the American Medical Association Opinion by misconstruing the text. Stahl and Emmanuel conflate declining to provide a particular kind of *treatment* with refusing to treat a particular kind of *patient*. To conscientiously object to a particular kind of treatment like abortion is not ethically equivalent to conscientiously objecting to a particular kind of person like women. A doctor might decline to provide abortion but continue to treat the patient and care for her in a variety of ways. Stahl and Emmanuel claim that the American Medical Association "permits physicians to refuse to treat patients who are seeking care,"[11] but this assertion is not to be found in the American Medical Association Opinion. The quotation cited by Stahl and Emmanuel from American Medical Association Opinion 1.1.2 addresses the refusal to provide particular *treatments*, not the refusal to treat particular *patients*. The legal and professional protection of the conscience rights of physicians has nothing to do with refusal to have women (or anyone else) as patients. Stahl and Emmanuel construct a contradiction only by misconstruing the AMA Opinion.

Even Stahl and Emmanuel concede that the professional obligations of physicians do not always trump their self-interest. "This obligation is not unlimited, but exceptions are reserved for cases in which there are substantial risks of permanent injury or death."[12] In fact, since conscience protections against being forced to perform abortions now exist, Stahl and Emmanuel are mistaken in claiming that exceptions are reserved by the professional codes only to cases of the risk of death and permanent injury.

Moreover, the exceptions in cases of risk of death or permanent injury lend support to conscience protections. Socrates taught that it is better to suffer harm than to do it.[13] Moral heroes through the centuries have lived according to this principle. Thomas More, Dietrich Bonhoeffer, Gandhi, Martin Luther King Jr., and Nelson Mandela were willing to suffer, and even to die, rather than violate their consciences. Like them, many people of goodwill would rather die than intentionally kill an innocent human being. If Kant is right that conscience is an unconditional command, then there can never be any interest whatsoever that trumps the demands of conscience. If it is worse to do harm than to suffer harm, health care workers' interests in not violating their consciences are maximally strong, indeed stronger even than their interests in avoiding death. Thus, even given Stahl and Emmanuel's stringent interpretation of the primacy of patient's interest, health care workers should be protected from violating their consciences. If the mere risk of permanent injury justifies putting the interest of the physician ahead of the interest of a patient, how much more would a certain harm to ethical integrity justify protecting health care professionals?

A final trouble with Stahl and Emmanuel's case against conscience is that there are many justifications of conscience protections for health care workers that do not depend upon appeal to conscience protections for those serving in the military. Stahl and Emmanuel make no reference to these arguments, nor do they even try to show that the analogy to conscience protections in the military is the *only* grounds used to justify conscience protections in health care. So even if Stahl and Emmanuel were successful in showing the disanalogy between military service and medical service, their case against conscience protections for health care workers leaves these other justifications for protecting the conscience rights of health care professionals untouched.[14]

Precisely speaking, what is at issue in this debate is not the interest of the patient in getting an abortion set against the interest of the doctor in not providing an abortion. Rather, the question is: Should a patient be able to force a particular doctor to perform an abortion? The right to get an abortion (from someone) is not at issue. In the United States, approximately one million abortions take place each year. Abortion is one of the most common surgeries performed in the United States, so current conscience protections have not led to an end to the practice of abortion. So at issue is not the right to get an abortion from someone who is willing to provide one but whether a patient should be able to force a particular health care professional to provide an abortion.

So let us consider a particular health care professional. What are the practical implications of the Stahl-Emmanuel rejection of conscience rights? Imagine you are a fifty-year-old Muslim gynecologist named Okina Makenzua who emigrated from Nigeria and now works in Los Angeles. You are also the mother of three children whom you support on your income alone. Despite living in a large metropolitan city, you are, as far as you know, the only female Nigerian Muslim gynecologist in the area. You make special efforts to serve the immigrant Muslim community. Likewise, Nigerian Muslim women make special efforts to come to you because you share their language, culture, and faith. They trust you, and you establish superb mutual understanding because of your shared background with your patients. Suddenly, the Stahl-Emmanuel constraint is imposed on you: provide abortions or get out of medicine. You feel you are too old and do not have the time and money to go back and learn another medical specialty like radiology. Your children and your ethnic community depend upon you in unique ways. In Los Angeles, there are dozens and dozens of abortion providers, but because you do not provide abortions you are suddenly forced out of your profession.

Who does Stahl-Emmanuel rule benefit? It directly and gravely harms Dr. Makenzua and her children. It harms the local Muslim community, who is deprived of a physician with a wonderful rapport with the recent immigrants. The Stahl-Emmanuel restriction does not even benefit women seeking abortions, since they already have dozens of abortion providers in the area and they lose the services of Dr. Makenzua, who is now no longer available to provide gynecological exams, or pap smears, or anything else. The Stahl-Emmanuel rule imposes severe and certain costs without proportional benefit.

If the US military had forced Private Doss out of military service, many men would have lost their lives on Hacksaw Ridge. If the Stahl-Emmanuel rule forces Dr. Makenzua and health care professionals like her out of medical service, she will suffer and we will all, directly or indirectly, suffer. Banning Private Doss and banning Dr. Makenzua from service are wrong for the same reason. Conscientious objection in military service and in medical service benefits not just conscientious objectors but all whom they serve.

Sixteen

Should Conscientiously Objecting Institutions Cover Elective Abortion in Their Insurance Plans?

SHOULD CATHOLIC UNIVERSITIES COVER ELECTIVE ABORTION IN THEIR insurance for employees?[1] This reflection considers the ethics of Catholic institutions choosing (where an institution is not legally obligated to cover elective abortion in its health insurance) to cover elective abortion in insurance, using the situation at Loyola Marymount University as a case study for one approach.

The LMU Board of Trustees decided the following: "We believe that the right to life and dignity for every human being is a fundamental part of Catholic beliefs (all other rights flow from this primary right to life and dignity), and that this vision needs to be evidenced in LMU's policies and procedures. Thus, the Board decided that LMU's principal insurance plans in 2014 will not provide coverage for elective abortions."[2] However, the LMU board also added that "a Third Party Administrator (TPA)-managed plan will be available. The TPA will be selected very shortly in order to facilitate an alternative. The TPA-managed plan will cover elective abortions, for which an employee will pay a slightly higher premium."[3]

169

Faculty and staff in favor of including abortion as part of the standard insurance argued that respect for the consciences of others in the diverse LMU community meant that LMU should include elective abortion in its insurance coverage. However, respect for the conscientious judgment of others does not require acting to facilitate people making choices that accord with these judgments. Respect for conscience involves refraining from manipulating, coercing, or otherwise attempting to force people to change their beliefs, but it does not involve cooperating, facilitating, or aiding others in carrying out actions based on their beliefs. Respect for conscience does not mean facilitating the choices of those with whom we disagree in conscience.

Employees in favor of including abortion coverage as part of the primary insurance also argue that many non-Catholics and dissenting Catholics work at LMU, so the university should not force these employees to adhere to Catholic teaching and "chill" their free speech on the abortion issue. However, all LMU employees enjoy freedom of religion, and therefore no LMU employee is forced to adhere to Catholic beliefs or practices. LMU employees can and do advocate for abortion rights, as was evident in the 189 some faculty and staff who signed a petition to the board urging the inclusion of abortion in insurance. In addition to not forcing employees to accept Catholic teaching, LMU also does nothing whatsoever to prevent faculty or staff from choosing elective abortion. Individuals working at LMU can choose (and may have chosen) to get abortions. Abortion is a legal right in the United States, but this legal right does not create legal or moral duties for others to pay for or otherwise facilitate abortion. In a similar way, a person's right to free speech is not violated if the university refuses to make that person a commencement speaker, pay for his or her books to be published, or let him or her address the incoming first-year students.

Unfortunately, the board's decision includes making available insurance coverage for elective abortion through a third party. This is morally problematic. Arranging for a third party to carry out an injustice for you does nothing to change your ethical responsibility for that injustice. Indeed, arranging for a third party to carry out an act of injustice is itself an act of injustice.

The board took a strong stand in the first part of their decision. In the second part of their decision, this strong stand was undermined. They decided to make available a third party to facilitate what they themselves view as an injustice against the dignity of the human person. What the board took away with their right hand they gave with their left. We consider abortion abhorrent, yet we have decided to facilitate it via a third party.

Bioethicist Roberto Dell'Oro offered a defense of the board's decision.[4] He correctly noted that "first, on strict Catholic grounds, one can never justify the choice of 'elective abortion.' The direct cooperation, therefore, of a Catholic university with its employees/students thus choosing is unacceptable. To tolerate the free choice of individuals is, of course, one thing; another is for a Catholic University to provide the conditions for that choice to successfully take place."[5] I would add that it is not simply a matter of "strict Catholic grounds" but also a matter of fundamental justice that persons of goodwill, regardless of faith, can understand and accept. Innocent human beings, both prenatally and postnatally, deserve our respect and care. I also agree with Dell'Oro that, illicit and unjust, "Proximate cooperation would take place were the University to offer coverage for 'elective abortion' through its health care carriers" and that remote material cooperation in wrongdoing is sometimes permissible.[6]

However, our agreement is not yet complete. Dell'Oro writes, "The University has chosen to eliminate coverage for abortion and to allow a third party administrator managed plan to establish arrangements for abortion coverage without using LMU dollars to pay for this additional coverage." This statement is not as accurate as it could be. "To allow" suggests that LMU is a passive, noninvolved spectator of someone else providing abortion coverage. In fact, LMU itself is arranging, facilitating, and making available the third-party administrator managed plan providing elective abortion coverage. LMU dollars, LMU time, and LMU efforts were used in order to arrange, facilitate, and make available the third-party administrator managed-plan coverage—a coverage that was chosen precisely because it includes elective abortion.

Given these facts, Dell'Oro is mistaken that this arrangement "provides the University with sufficient 'distance' from the choice of elective abortion."[7] Unfortunately, such arrangements do not make a moral difference. LMU's providing the third-party administrator managed plan is like someone saying, "Since I think abortion is intentional killing, I won't drive you to the abortion clinic, but I'll arrange for my brother to drive you to the clinic if you pay him a few bucks." This arrangement does not create clean hands. In neither case is the cooperation "remote."

Dell'Oro holds that "LMU's solution stands between two extremes: the dogmatic imposition of values on personal conscience and decision making, on the one hand; the identification, without further qualification, of freedom of conscience and freedom of choice, on the other."[8] This way of characterizing the issue is problematic. The decision not to cover elective abortion in insurance in no way imposes values on conscience and decision making. In the past few years, in which LMU covered elective abortions, this did not coerce, manipulate, or otherwise attempt to force people to change their conscientious beliefs about abortion. To refuse to cover abortion is not an attempt to coerce, manipulate, or impose values on people's consciences. And if LMU had chosen not to provide a third-party administrator managed plan (as President Fr. Michael Engh did at Santa Clara University), again no one's conscience would have been coerced. Just as we can respect the conscientious political beliefs of others but also not cooperate in facilitating their support of their political party, so too the university could respect people who claim the label "prochoice" and not facilitate their choice to abort. In all three possibilities, LMU employees have every legal right to get abortions and conscientiously hold any view they would like about abortion.

In portraying LMU's position as an intermediary between two opposing extreme views, the implicit premise is that virtue lies in the mean. But, as Aristotle pointed out in the *Nicomachean Ethics*, not all actions admit of a virtuous mean.[9] Among the actions that do not admit of a virtuous mean is killing innocent human beings or formally cooperating in killing innocent human beings.

Dell'Oro writes, "Consistency suggests that the ethos of pluralism, of respect for diversity of moral and religious sensibilities, of openness and dialogue, so clearly treasured by our University, cannot be abruptly bracketed in matters of health care decisions, including matters of reproductive choice. Respect for conscience demands that whatever policy LMU adopts, it sees it as an articulation, rather than a suspension, of that very ethos."[10] Respect for conscience and diversity is a two-way street. If prochoice employees at LMU ask that the university respect their consciences and not force them to act against their consciences, then these same employees should show respect for the conscience of those who wish to maintain LMU as "institutionally devoted to Roman Catholicism" in its practices.

It is actually prochoice employees who are seeking to impose their values on others by forcing them to cooperate in actions that LMU as an institution believes to be unjust.

Finally, Dell'Oro writes, "The commitment to a position that enhances both the life of the unborn and the health of women warrants, in my opinion, the policy adopted by LMU: the exclusion of direct coverage for elective abortion by the University, with the provision of a TPA for those who want to maintain open for themselves the space of free choice."[11] I do not agree with the assertion that elective abortion enhances women's health. By definition, elective abortion is optional and is not therefore necessary for the life or health of the mother. Indeed, in many cases, abortion itself seriously damages the physical and psychological health of women. As the Jesuit statement "Standing for the Unborn" put it, "To be pro-life is to be prowoman. Because we support women, we oppose abortion."[12] Finally, "free choice" is not at issue. Subsidizing, supporting, and cooperating with choices to kill are the issue.

Another defense of offering a third-party administrator managed plan appeals to the principle of double effect or double-effect reasoning. According to this argument, the action itself of providing insurance that covers abortion is not intrinsically evil as a means, nor is providing such insurance evil as an end. Abortion itself, if it happens, is merely a foreseen but not intended effect of the action of providing insurance, an action that has two effects—one bad (facilitating abortion) and one good (facilitating genuine health care). Double-effect reasoning would seem to cover this case. The (possible) bad side effect is that someone is enabled to get an abortion. The good effect is that it provides something desired by employees. So, since the evil is not intended, the action would be justified by double-effect reasoning.

I am skeptical that double-effect reasoning justifies the decision at hand. In this case, the third-party administrator managed plan was chosen precisely because it covered abortion, not out of ignorance. The evil effect is intended. The desired effect of pleasing faculty and staff wanting abortion coverage is accomplished only by deliberately including abortion coverage. It would seem that the first principle of double-effect reasoning is violated, namely that the act itself is not evil. The act of choosing some package deal precisely in order to facilitate an intrinsically evil act is itself intrinsically evil. Such a case is not merely material cooperation with evil, but in virtue of choosing the package precisely because it includes the evil, it is formal cooperation in evil, which is always wrong.

Even if the evil of abortion were merely a side effect, it is still not clear that providing such coverage would be justified by double-effect reasoning. The fourth condition of double-effect reasoning is that there is a proportionate or commensurate reason for allowing the evil effect. In order to determine whether it is reasonable to allow an evil effect in order to secure the good effect, it is important to consider the gravity of the evil effect and the good effect. Imagine a pregnant woman taking aspirin to relieve a minor headache. She knows that taking the aspirin will cause her child to have Reye's syndrome and therefore be permanently and seriously disabled. Double-effect reasoning would not justify her choice, even though her intention in taking the aspirin was not to harm the baby. The reason is that the evil of the child having Reye's syndrome is so much more serious than the evil of suffering a minor headache. Similarly, the evil of choosing abortion and the evil of an innocent child losing his or her life are very serious evils. The good of appeasing faculty and staff who feel aggravated that the Catholic university does not cover abortion is not commensurate with the evil of abortion.

Furthermore, another factor to be considered in coming to a conclusion about whether a proportionate reason is present is whether alternative ways of securing the good in question are available. Let us say in the case of the headache just described that instead of taking aspirin the woman took acetaminophen. Both would eliminate the headache. If alternatives exist for securing the good that do not bring about the bad side effect, these alternatives should be chosen rather than the alternative that does bring about the bad side effect.

In this case, were there any other ways of helping employees understand that LMU values them as employees and cares about diversity in the faculty and staff? It seems there are multiple ways, such as having administrators give speeches affirming rights to free speech and freedom of belief, explaining how the policy does not take away anyone's legal rights to abortion, and providing extra funding for addressing the concerns of aggrieved parties on campus. The university could have sought these goods without providing abortion insurance.

Another defense of LMU's action points out that the prior insurance benefit provided abortion as part of the overall package of health care. This was morally permissible: the cooperation in the wrongdoing of someone choosing abortion would be remote, since it was removed in time, space, and by human choice from the actual decision to choose abortion. The new third-party administrator managed plan is even more remote, since now the extra coverage is not paid for by the university and an employee must explicitly opt into the plan. In both cases, the remote material justification for the evil is justified by the goods of providing supposedly just compensation for employees in terms of health insurance.

The trouble with this defense of a third-party administrator managed plan in this situation is that once abortion can be excluded from coverage, abortion no longer becomes part of a "package deal" and an ethically different situation exists. It is one thing to drive a bus that just happens to go past an abortion clinic, even if you know some people will ride the bus to get an abortion. It is quite another to choose to drive a bus precisely because it goes past an abortion clinic so that those who ride the bus to get an abortion will have someone to give them a ride. If abortion were just one part of the package deal, if no alternative health insurance coverage without abortion were available, the choice of providing health insurance (that as part of the package also included abortion) could be justified as remote material cooperation. By contrast, the choice to set up a third-party administrator managed plan precisely with the intention that the third-party administrator managed plan cover elective abortion is no longer remote cooperation, since it is no longer simply a "package deal." When the third-party administrator managed plan is set up in this situation, elective abortion coverage is not regrettably tolerated as part of the package of providing health insurance. Rather, the choice of the third-party administrator managed plan is motivated precisely by the inclusion of elective abortion. Indeed, a third-party administrator managed plan that did not include elective abortion coverage would not have been chosen. So the new policy does not virtually eliminate but rather increases the cooperation with evil in comparison to the older plan.

Another argument in favor of providing insurance for abortion is that the lowest-paid employees—those who are in most "need" of abortion— would be most adversely affected by removing abortion coverage. Justice demands that those who are the least well-off be especially taken into account.

But those who are least well-off and most vulnerable are not the lowest-paid employees but rather the prenatal human beings who may lose their lives. Further, this argument presupposes that getting an abortion is actually beneficial. But if abortion is unjust, it cannot be truly beneficial to the one who gets the abortion. Indeed, making it more difficult for others to do an unjust thing is not itself an injustice done to them but rather a service to them.

It is indeed possible (as the case of Thomas Aquinas College shows) not to provide insurance for elective abortion at all. Institutions that are consistent in embracing their mission can follow this example.

Seventeen

Is It Ethically Permissible to Separate Conjoined Twins?

THE PSEUDONYMS "JODIE" AND "MARY" WERE GIVEN TO CONJOINED twins from Malta who were born with serious health problems, including the fact that Jodie's heart pumped blood for both of them. As the twins grew, doctors foresaw with certainty that Jodie's heart could not sustain pumping blood for both girls. They thus advised surgically separating the girls in order to save Jodie's life. Questions arose: Is it ethically permissible to separate the twins, foreseeing with certainty that the separation will end Mary's life? Does the separation constitute mutilation of one person in order to save another? Is there a duty to perform the surgical separation even against the parents' wishes? British courts and ethicists around the world weighed in on questions such as these as well as the legal implications. The case of Jodie and Mary, and many other medical interventions on conjoined twins, raise important questions. To adjudicate the ethics of separating conjoined twins, it is necessary first to have at least some implicit answer to a variety of other questions. The first of these, both logically and in importance, is the moral status of conjoined twins.

CONJOINED TWINS AND HUMAN DIGNITY

Do conjoined twins have basic human dignity? Are conjoined twins one (or two) of us? Krzysztof Kobylarz explores the causes and kinds of conjoined twins as understood by the ancient writers Democritus, Empedocles, and Aristotle, as well as writers in the late twentieth century.[1] They did not all recognize the inherent dignity of conjoined twins. Kobylarz includes twenty-six drawings and photographs of conjoined twins united at the head, chest, rump, and in virtually every other combination imaginable. Many of the pictures are shocking, even grotesque. It is easy to see the origins of the ancient dehumanizing habit of describing conjoined twins as "monsters." Unfortunately, Kobylarz perpetuates this dehumanizing tradition by speaking of one conjoined twin who was dependent on a sibling as "a parasite foetus." "Despite the doctors' efforts," writes Kobylarz, "the child died shortly after separation from the parasite."[2]

It is hard to imagine words more likely to contribute to dehumanization than speaking of an innocent human being as a "parasite fetus." As John Finnis said at the event "Open Hearts, Open Minds, and Fair-Minded Words: A Conference on Life and Choice in the Abortion Debate," held at Princeton University, it is important to use our language with care lest we dehumanize fellow human beings:

> About the moral status of the phrase "the fetus," I will just say this. As used in . . . [non-]medical contexts, it is offensive, dehumanizing, prejudicial, manipulative. Used in this [non-medical] context, exclusively and in preference to the alternatives, it is an F-word, to go with the J-word, and other such words we know of, which have or had an acceptable meaning in a proper context but became in wider use the symbol of subjection to the prejudices and preferences of the more powerful. It's not a fair word, and it does not suggest an open heart. Those of you who have an open mind or a fair heart may wish to listen to every speaker at this conference, and see whether they are willing to speak, at least sometimes, of the unborn child or unborn baby, and to do so without scare quotes or irony.[3]

It is wrong, both theoretically and practically, to use language to dehumanize human beings. Dehumanizing language is theoretically wrong because it is untruthful. Human beings who are conjoined twins are no more and no less human than any other human beings. Dehumanizing language is practically wrong because it contributes to rationalizations for treating human beings as less than human.

So let us not speak of conjoined twins as "fetuses," or "parasites," or "monsters"; for such ways of speaking may lead us and others to begin to forget that people are equal in basic dignity despite any disability. Although some people have denied this basic equality to human conjoined twins, for reasons discussed earlier in this book, all human beings, conjoined or not, are created equal and endowed with inalienable rights.

Although they were not innocent of using the language of "monster" for conjoined twins, Catholic writers, in both theory and practice, recognized the humanity of human beings with fused bodies. Irven Resnick explores the fascinating way in which patristic and medieval Scholastics dealt with the topic of conjoined twins, such as this passage from Augustine's *De civitate Dei*: "Some years ago, quite within my own memory, a man was born in the East, doubled in his upper members, but single in his lower ones. For he had two heads, two chests, four hands, but one belly and two feet like one man; and he lived so long that rumor [of him] drew many people to see him."[4]

Much of the medieval debate concerned the causes of conjoined twins, a topic explored by Albert the Great. Resnick chronicles how medieval Scholastics, often spurred by questions posed at quodlibetal sessions in the universities, also sought to understand how the sacraments applied to conjoined twins. Concerning baptism, the consensus view seemed to have been that, if there are two heads and two hearts, then there are two souls, and hence there is need for two baptisms. However, other conjoined body parts, such as additional fingers or toes, were not viewed as constituting additional people. But questions remained.

Part of the medieval dispute centered on whether the head or the heart was the principal organ of the body sufficient for identifying an individual person. Henry of Ghent argued that, if there were two heads but only one heart, then just one baptism was required because the second head was just an appendage of one human body.[5] On the other hand, if there were two hearts, Henry concluded, "it is necessary to assert that such a monster has two rational souls, with the result that they are truly two persons and two human beings."[6] Other Scholastics argued that two heads were enough, even with a single shared heart, to constitute two persons. For example, John Pecham argued that each head should be baptized and that, if there was some question, after the first baptism the other baptism could be conditionally made: "If you are not already baptized, I baptize you in the name of the Father, and of the Son, and of the Holy Spirit."[7] The view that eventually prevailed in the Catholic tradition was that there should be as many baptisms as there were heads.[8] These discussions of the sacramental validity of baptism underscore that, in the Catholic tradition, conjoined twins are persons with human dignity. I believe this same conclusion can be defended without appeal to revelation or theological tradition. In any case, my remarks on the ethics of separating conjoined twins will presuppose the truth of this view.

CONJOINED TWINS AND INTENTIONAL KILLING

If one twin will certainly die from the procedure, is separating conjoined twins intentional killing? Put simply, is it murder? A sound answer to the question of separation depends upon both relevant biological details and philosophical considerations. As a matter of biology, conjoined twins are found in a wide variety of conditions and are often classified on the basis of their point of union.[9]

For example, thoracopagus twins are joined at the chest, omphalopagus twins are joined at the abdomen, and craniopagus twins are joined at the head. Another classification is as symmetrical—both twins well developed—or asymmetrical—one twin well formed and the other not. In heteropagus twinning, one twin is dependent for life on the other. One can also imagine a case in which both twins are dependent on each other—for example, one has a functioning heart and the other has a functioning liver.

The point of joining does not seem morally significant insofar as in some cases of, say, twins joined at the head, the twins might be superficially joined and thereby easily separated, restoring natural bodily integrity to both and endangering the life and well-being of neither. On the other hand, in some instances of twins joined at the rump, the two might be so profoundly fused that to separate them would risk or even necessarily bring about death to one or both. What is ethically relevant is not the site of conjunction but the likely effects of both leaving the twins conjoined and of separating them. Here we can distinguish a range of cases based on various factors. One factor is whether both twins will be benefited, just one twin will be benefited, or both twins will be harmed. Another factor is the likely harm involved, ranging from death at one extreme through serious disability to minor disability all the way to normal health. Another factor is the likely benefits, ranging from saving someone's life and restoring someone to normal health to, on the other, extremely negligible benefits or no benefit. Yet another factor is the likelihood of various harms and benefits, ranging from certainty on one extreme to impossibility on the other.

Part of the difficulty in considering the case of conjoined twins ethically is that these factors will vary significantly from case to case. Even leaving aside the inherent medical difficulties in performing the surgical separation of profoundly conjoined twins, including difficulty in prognosticating what will happen if they are separated and if they are not, it is easy to imagine medical experts having sharply divided views about the likelihood of various harms and benefits.

Keeping all these difficulties in mind, it might be helpful to consider a range of situations. On the one extreme are cases in which both twins will benefit from separation. The ethics of separation in such cases is simple. If consent is given by adult conjoined twins, or if parental consent is given in the case of minor conjoined twins, it is permissible to separate the twins. If separating conjoined twins will not kill or injure either one, and both twins consent—or, in the case of twins unable to consent, there is rightful proxy consent—I can see no reason why their separation would be morally wrong. On the other extreme are cases in which neither twin benefits from separation. The answer is just as clear here that, if separation harms both twins, then it is impermissible. These are the easy cases. The hard cases are ones in which one twin will benefit and the other will be harmed in separation.

In the most ethically difficult cases, separating conjoined twins may be medically necessary to save one twin but will certainly kill the other. In such examples, not just possible harm but certain death awaits one twin even as the same separation benefits the other. Such was the case of Jodie and Mary. The heart and lungs most closely associated with Mary's body could not circulate blood for her, so oxygenated blood came by way of Jodie's heart and lungs. Physicians foresaw that Jodie's lungs and heart were incapable of sustaining long-term support for both girls. The choice facing the physicians, parents, and courts was whether to separate the girls. If the girls were not separated, they would both die. If they were separated, Jodie would likely survive but Mary would surely die. Is separating them intentional killing? Is unjoining them intentional mutilation? Is there an obligation to separate them?

The answer to such questions depends in part on the account of intention adopted. In contemporary discussion of natural law ethics, two accounts of intention have emerged: what might be called the "narrow view" and the "broad view." Advocates of the New Natural Law theory—such as John Finnis, Germain Grisez, and Joseph Boyle—argue for the narrow account of intention in which only those effects that are chosen as a means or as an end in an agent's proposed plan count as intended.[10] All other effects are merely foreseen. So a man who goes jogging does not intend to perspire or to wear out his running shoes. One could, of course, imagine some odd case in which the goal of his jogging was to wear out the shoes, since, say, he knew a much better pair of shoes was coming his way as soon as this pair was worn out. But normally, wearing out running shoes is not part of what is intended either as a means or as an end. Wearing out running shoes is *praeter intentionem.*

Advocates of classic natural law theory—such as Stephen Brock, Lawrence Dewan, and Kevin Flannery—argue that intention cannot be limited to effects chosen precisely as a means or end, but includes other effects as well.[11] The broad view holds that other effects must be included in the agent's intention: for example, those effects that are closely related, or are foreseen with certainty, or are part of the act as a reasonable person would understand the act, and so forth. Although they may disagree about what effects should be included as intended and on what grounds, the classic natural law theorists agree in rejecting the narrow view.

Both classic and new natural law advocates agree that counterfactual criteria for determining intention do not work. After all, in murder in order to cover a theft, the killer could truthfully say to his gagged and bound victim, "If there were any other way I could secure your silence about my theft, if only there were a pill you could take to erase your memory of this whole event, I would certainly spare your life. But since no such pill exists, I have to kill you to make sure that you don't reveal my identity." He then shoots her in the head, twice. If this is not intentional killing, then nothing is.

Aside from this agreement, much separates the broad and the narrow views of intention, including the proper interpretation of Thomas Aquinas, whether the new natural law theory is Cartesian in its account of intention, and whether the broad or narrow view best accounts for our intuitions about various concrete cases, such as, for example, craniotomy or the use of methotrexate to treat ectopic pregnancies. A full consideration of the arguments for and against the narrow view of intention falls outside the scope of this chapter. It will be enough to consider how these two views would approach the case of conjoined twins such as Jodie and Mary.

On the narrow view of intention, the separation of Jodie and Mary is not a case of intentional killing, since physicians separating the twins are not seeking Mary's death as a means or an end of their procedure. Yes, Mary's death will result from the procedure, but, like the prenatal death that occurs in the removal of a gravid cancerous uterus, her death is not intended as a means or an end. In both Mary's case and the case of removing a cancerous uterus early in pregnancy, the death of the human beings is a foreseen side effect—*praeter intentionem*, to use Aquinas's phrase—of a morally legitimate action.

On the broad account of intention, as understood by Matthew O'Brien and Robert Koons, the separation might seem to be intentional killing.[12] The doctors, in the case of Jodie and Mary, knew with full certainty that separation from Jodie would inevitably cause Mary's death. However, if the separation were understood as akin to the removal of a tubal pregnancy, the broad account might still be able to account for Mary's death as a side effect. About ectopic pregnancy, O'Brien and Koons write,

> In removing the tube the surgeon is not depriving the embryo of a condition that is sufficient for its survival, nor of a condition that is natural for the embryo at that point in its development, and the embryo doesn't have a claim on its mother to extend momentarily its

unnatural growth at the cost of her death. By removing the fallopian tube, the surgeon is removing an unnatural delayer of the child's death: he is not thereby causing, or even hastening her death, which is due to the absence of the supply of oxygen and nutrients from a placenta properly implanted in the womb. Removing the tube and removing the cancerous uterus are similar because both are targeted remedies of defective biological functioning.[13]

Similar reasoning could be used to justify the separation of Jodie and Mary. The conjunction of Jodie and Mary is an unnatural union. In separating them, the surgeons are not depriving Mary of a condition that is sufficient for her survival, nor of a condition that is natural for her in terms of human functioning, and she doesn't have a claim on Jodie to extend indefinitely their unnatural union at the cost of Jodie's death. By separating Mary and Jodie, the surgeon is removing an unnatural delayer of Mary's death. The surgeon is not thereby causing, or even hastening, Mary's death, which is due to the absence of sufficient oxygenated blood from her own malfunctioning heart. Separating Jodie and Mary and removing the ectopic pregnancy in a fallopian tube are similar, because both are targeted remedies of defective biological functioning in Jodie and the mother respectively. If this analysis is correct, then Jodie and Mary's separation would not be a case of intentional killing but a case of letting one die, even on a broad account of intention.

CONJOINED TWINS, MUTILATION, AND THE BENEFITS OF SURGERY

One objection to separating conjoined twins is that the separation is intentional mutilation and that mutilation is an intrinsically evil act. The separation of conjoined twins may not be killing—on either the narrow or the broad account of intention—but it is a surgical intervention that counts as mutilation.

But what exactly is mutilation? I propose for consideration the following definition: "Mutilation is the intentional destruction or removal of an organ (or other vital body part) that inhibits the function that the organ had or will likely have in maintaining the health of the one possessing the organ."[14] The question then becomes, whose organs are whose? In considering whether separating conjoined twins counts as mutilation, it is helpful to use M. Cathleen Kaveny's distinction between the Bodily Distinctiveness View and the Bodily Relatedness View. According to the former, medical facts are used to judge which organs belong to which twin. As much as possible, each body part is allotted to a specific twin, and "An organ would be deemed to be a 'shared' organ if and only if it was equally enmeshed with the relevant systems of both babies."[15] According to the Bodily Distinctiveness View, surgical separation seeks to bring to order the proper independence of each of the bodies. Assuming that the surgeons do not attempt the destruction or removal of organs inhibiting the health of either twin possessing the organ, the surgical intervention is not mutilation. Since the goal is to save the healthy twin, surgeons attempt to avoid mutilation for this twin. Since the weaker twin dies as a result of the surgery, mutilation is also not at issue, presuming that surgeons don't intentionally remove or inhibit this twin's organs and the twin dies as a side effect of being separated from the healthy twin.

By contrast, in the Bodily Relatedness View, organs that function for the good of both twins "belong" to both twins, even if the organ would clearly belong to one twin according to the Bodily Distinctiveness View: "The Bodily Relatedness View would contend that the complex, intertwined, two-in-one body that the twins share has its own integrity meriting our respect, precisely as the body of two-in-one."[16] According to the Bodily Relatedness View, both babies "have a rightful claim upon all essential organs, until it is proven otherwise. . . . An organ will be said to belong exclusively to one twin if and only if it does not provide essential support for the other."[17] However, if "both will be better off after the separation, then the procedure should be performed."[18] On the other hand, "If the surgery will not be beneficial to both, it will be unfair to the baby whose prospects are poorer unless the detriment to that baby is slight and the benefit to his or her twin considerable."[19]

If we apply this standard to cases such as Jodie and Mary, then the separation is still justified. The reason is that, although the surgery will not be beneficial to both, the detriment to the baby who dies is slight and the benefit to the other twin is considerable. But the healthier twin has a shot at a regular life span if and only if the separation takes place. Why claim that the detriment to the sicker baby is slight?

Death, of course, is enormously detrimental, but this side effect is certain no matter what decision is made. If the twins are not separated, the weaker twin will soon die. If the twins are separated, the weaker twin will soon die. It may be that the side effect of death comes sooner in one scenario than the other, but the slight difference in timing makes only a slight difference in terms of how detrimental the side effect is in comparison with how detrimental the same side effect would be if the surgery were not performed.

A difficulty with this argument is that it would not apply to all cases of conjoined twins where they cannot continue to live as conjoined, particularly cases in which there is no "weaker twin" who is doomed to die. Consider two twins, Sean and Troy, who are like Jodie and Mary but with an important twist: mutual interdependence. According to the Bodily Distinctiveness View, Sean uses Troy's heart and Troy uses Sean's lungs. Troy's heart cannot maintain circulation for both; nor can Sean's lungs. In this case, suppose there is no "weaker twin" doomed to die whether or not surgery is performed. Who should be saved?

In a case like this, supposing for the sake of argument there is no medical reason to think one has a greater chance at life than the other, a decision should be made on the basis of chance, like flipping a coin. If both twins cannot be saved, then it is licit to try to save one who can be saved, even if the other twin will die as a side effect of the operation. It would not, however, be obligatory in all cases to separate such twins, for such surgeries can be considered extraordinary means of saving life.

QUESTIONS OF CONSENT

Another important issue is that of consent to the separation surgery. Let us pose, but leave aside, a vexing case. What should be done if one adult conjoined twin wishes for separation and the other does not want separation? In cases of profoundly conjoined twins, it could be, as in the case of Jodie and Mary, that both will die if they are not separated, but one can survive and the other will die more quickly if they are separated. In such cases, as well as others, what should be done if the twins, both consenting adults, disagree with each other? I leave this good question here unanswered. On the other hand, if two adult conjoined twins, capable of giving informed consent, have been informed of all the relevant risks and benefits of the separation, they may licitly choose to be separated.

Let's assume that informed consent by the twins cannot be given because they are too young. If separation is not necessary to save the life of one twin, may parents or guardians give consent based on the standard of presumed consent? Kaveny argues that they may:

> Even if Jodie's connection to Mary does not kill her, it gravely impedes her flourishing. It will prevent her from ever walking, and even from sitting up properly. It will impede her participation in forms of life that are greatly facilitated by bodily distinctness, such as marriage. On the analogy that sees Jodie as providing life support to Mary, one would argue that Jodie has no duty to do so under circumstances that will gravely hamper her own flourishing. Her parents have no right to expect her to sacrifice her own bodily integrity in order to support her sister's failing heart and lungs, any more than they would have a right to expect one non-conjoined twin to donate an organ to save the other's life, if she would sacrifice the expectation of a normal, independent life by making such a donation.[20]

This argument hinges on the assumption that being a conjoined twin gravely impedes flourishing. Is this assumption justified? What is meant here by *flourishing*?

The psychologist Martin Seligman defines *flourishing* in terms of positive emotion, engagement with life, positive relationships, meaning in making a contribution to something larger, and achievement/accomplishment of personal goals (PERMA). Conjoined twins can have all the elements of PERMA. If we think of flourishing in terms of loving God and neighbor, again the bodily connection of conjoined twins does not necessarily undermine flourishing. If we turn to the lived experience of conjoined twins, they often report that they enjoy their condition and would not want to be separated. People often think that the adult life of conjoined twins would be an unbearable misery and that twins are better off separated even at the risk of death or severe disability. In fact, in most cases, adult conjoined twins do not want to be separated: "Many singletons, especially surgeons, find it inconceivable that life is worth living as a conjoined twin, inconceivable that one would not be willing to risk all— mobility, reproductive ability, the life of one or both twins—to try for separation";[21] but an exhaustive examination of the research finds "the desire to remain together to be so widespread among communicating conjoined twins as to be practically universal."[22] Not even the goods of marriage are necessarily excluded for conjoined twins. Famously, Siamese twins Chang and Eng produced twenty-one children in their marriage to two sisters.

But perhaps not a physical but a moral constraint blocks the marriage of conjoined twins. Are conjoined twins eligible for marriage? May conjoined twins give valid consent to enter into the sacrament of matrimony as understood by the Catholic Church? Fourteenth-century Parisian master Eustache de Grandcourt saw a serious difficulty, at least in cases of conjoined twins with two heads capable of giving consent but only one body below the head. Eustache posed the objection that, for such persons, marriage was impossible. A wife may be sexually intimate only with her husband. In the case of conjoined male twins, however, she would be intimate not only with the twin whom she consented to marry but also with the other twin in virtue of the twins sharing only "one instrument of generation."[23] So, in consummating the marriage, she and her brother-in-law would simultaneously be committing adultery. On the other hand, if she attempted to consent to marry both twins, this too would be impossible, for monogamy rather than bigamy is the Christian form of marriage.

Despite raising this objection, Eustache concluded that conjoined persons may indeed get married because they have been given everything necessary for marriage. They can give consent and consummate the marriage. Nature does not act in vain.

There is, perhaps, another way to resolve the adultery-bigamy dilemma. Consider Chad and Peter, conjoined twins having two heads but just one body below the head. Chad wants to marry Laura, Laura wants to marry Chad, and both are otherwise eligible to marry. Christian marriage excludes bigamy, so Chad and Peter cannot both consent to marry Laura, and Laura may consent only to marry either Chad or Peter. Chad and Laura exchange marriage vows—so far, so good.

However, in consummating the marriage, do Laura and her brother-in-law Peter commit adultery? At least on some accounts of intention, Laura and Peter are not necessarily intending to join themselves together in a sexual way. The sexual union of Peter and Laura is a foreseen side effect rather than something either one necessarily chooses. The sin of adultery must be something *chosen*, not just something that happens to one's body without choice. By similar reasoning, a married woman who is raped does not commit adultery, even though she is physically united to someone other than her husband. Since the consummation of the marriage need not involve adultery, conjoined twins with two heads but only one body may enter into marriage—an unusual marriage, but a marriage nonetheless.

Conjoined twins can enjoy the goods of marriage, friendship, knowledge, life, and so forth. Indeed, most adult conjoined twins report that they do enjoy life and do not wish to be separated even if they could. If this research on the preferences of adult conjoined twins is accurate, then perhaps we should recognize that there is no presumed consent for separation unless separation is needed to save life. If interest is construed subjectively and if most conjoined twins prefer to remain conjoined when given the choice, then the presumed subjective interest of conjoined twins who cannot consent would suggest not separating them.

Is it in their interests to be separated if their interests are objectively construed? It may not be, particularly if death or severe injury is likely for one or both. On the other hand, it may be that one or both will die if not separated; so, in cases like Jodie and Mary, it would be objectively in the interest of the only twin who can survive to be separated.

In such cases, M. Cathleen Kaveny rightly notes a problematic aspect of parental consent to the surgery.[24] Following Aquinas, she notes that there can be a conflict between parties in which *both* are doing God's will for them but they are doing opposite things. Aquinas gives the example of a widow who wishes her husband to be spared the death penalty. It is good and right for her to do so. It is also good and right for the minister of justice to carry out the just punishment— just, at least, according to Aquinas. Another example is a priest, who may not carry out public justice in killing malefactors, and the minister of justice, who has an obligation to do so.

In a similar way, given their role as parents, Jodie and Mary's mother and father acted rightly in not authorizing the surgical separation of the girls because the separation would not benefit, but only harm, Mary. Kaveny notes, "It is 'unfitting' for parents to authorize or cooperate with the physical or psychological treatment of a child in a way that will bring that child no benefit, but only harm."[25] But what is unfitting for parents to do to their own children, in light of the special concern parents owe to their own children, may be fitting for others, like judges, to do in light of their concern for the good of the life of citizens. The judges, in ordering the separation, also acted rightly in preserving vulnerable human life, even at the cost of losing another vulnerable human life as a side effect of the surgery.

CONCLUSION

In summary, it is not necessarily intentional killing to separate conjoined twins, even if one will certainly die from the operation. If adult conjoined twins give informed consent, it is permissible for them to be separated. If conjoined twins are too young or too infirm to give consent, parents or guardians may give presumed consent in cases in which separation is necessary to secure the continued life of the twin that can survive. In cases in which separation is done in order to improve "quality of life," separation is probably not justified on the basis of presumed consent, since most adult conjoined twins do not want to be separated.

Acknowledgments

The author would like to thank the editors and publishers of the following journals for their permission to reproduce the following materials. Chapter 1 and chapter 4 originally appeared at *Public Discourse: The Journal of the Witherspoon Institute*, www.thepublicdiscourse.com. Chapters 2, 3, 5, 6, 9, and 14–16 originally appeared in the *National Catholic Bioethics Quarterly*. Chapters 7 and 8 appeared first in the pages of *Bioethics*. Chapter 10 is reprinted from an essay originally entitled, "Married Love, God's Plan, and the Good of Children" in *Humanae Vitae, Fifty Years Later*, edited by Theresa Notare (Washington, DC: The Catholic University of America Press, 2019). Chapter 11, with co-author Robert P. George, appears in *Assisted Death and Human Dignity*, ed. Sebastian Muders (New York: Oxford University Press, 2017). Chapter 12 was originally, "Against Euthanasia for Children: A Response to Bovens," *Journal of Medical Ethics* 42, no.1 (2016): 57–58. Chapter 17 first appeared as "Is It Ethically Permissible to Separate Conjoined Twins? Murder, Mutilation, and Consent" in *Contemporary Controversies in Catholic Bioethics*, edited by Jason T. Eberl, Philosophy and Medicine Series (Springer, 2017).

Finally, I also owe an enormous debt of gratitude for support in writing sections of this book to the James Madison Program of Princeton University.

Notes

Chapter 1.   *Is Speciesism a Form of Prejudice?*

1. Singer's words as cited by Shelly Kagan, "What's Wrong with Speciesism?," Society of Applied Philosophy Annual Lecture 2015, *Journal of Applied Philosophy* 33.1 (February 2016): 1, doi: 10.1111/japp.12164.

2. Ibid., 3.

3. Ibid., 8.

4. Ibid., 9.

5. Ibid., 10.

6. Thomas Aquinas, *Summa contra gentiles* 3.112.1, ed. and trans. Vernon J. Bourke (Notre Dame, IN: University of Notre Dame Press, 1975). See, too, his *Commentary on the Sentences of Peter Lombard* 44.1.3 ad 1.

7. Immanuel Kant, *Grounding for the Metaphysics of Morals* 2.429, trans. James E. Ellington (Indianapolis: Hackett, 1993).

8. Sherif Girgis, "Equality and Moral Worth in Natural Law Ethics and Beyond," *American Journal of Jurisprudence* 59.2 (2014): 143–62.

9. Thomas Aquinas, *Summa theologiae* II-II, 26, 6, trans. Fathers of the English Dominican Province (Notre Dame, IN: Christian Classics, 1947).

10. Thomas Aquinas, *Sententia libri Politicorum* 1.1.32, trans. Ernest L. Fortin and Peter D. O'Neill as *Commentary on Aristotle's "Politics"* (New York: Free Press of Glencoe, 1963), https://dhspriory.org/thomas/Politics.htm.

11. Kant, *Grounding* 2.429 (trans. Ellington).

12. David DeGrazia, "Modal Personhood and Moral Status: A Reply to Kagan's Proposal," *Journal of Applied Philosophy* 33.1 (February 2016): 22–25, esp. 24.

13. Ibid., 24–25.

14. Peter Singer, "Why Speciesism Is Wrong: A Response to Kagan," *Journal of Applied Philosophy* 33.1 (February 2016): 32, doi: 10.1111/japp.12165.

15. Ibid.

Chapter 2. *What Is Dignity?*

1. Glenn Hughes, "The Concept of Dignity in the Universal Declaration of Human Rights," *Journal of Religious Ethics* 39.1 (March 2011): 8.

2. Bharat Ranganathan, "Should Inherent Human Dignity Be Considered Intrinsically Heuristic?," *Journal of Religious Ethics* 42.4 (2014): 770–75.

3. Daniel Sulmasy, "The Varieties of Human Dignity: A Logical and Conceptual Analysis," *Medicine, Health Care, and Philosophy* 16.4 (2013): 937–44.

4. Ibid., 943.

5. Sherif Girgis, "Equality and Moral Worth in Natural Law Ethics and Beyond," *American Journal of Jurisprudence* 59.2 (2014): 143–62.

6. Carlo Leget, "Analyzing Dignity: A Perspective from the Ethics of Care," *Medicine, Health Care and Philosophy* 16.4 (November 2013): 945–52.

7. Ibid., 947.

8. Ibid., 949.

9. Ibid.

10. Colin Bird, "Dignity as a Moral Concept," *Social Philosophy and Policy* 30.1–2 (January 2013): 150–76.

11. Alan Gewirth, *Self-Fulfillment* (Princeton, NJ: Princeton University Press, 2009), 168–69.

12. Ibid., 169.

13. Leget, "Analyzing Dignity," 949.

Chapter 3. *Should We Make Children with Three (or More) Parents?*

1. Daniela Cutas et al., "Artificial Gametes: Perspectives of Geneticists, Ethicists, and Representatives of Potential Users," *Medicine, Health Care, and Philosophy* 17.3 (August 2014): 343.

2. Ibid.

3. Ibid., 341.

4. César Palacios-González, John Harris, and Giuseppe Testa, "Multiplex Parenting: IVG and the Generations to Come," *Journal of Medical Ethics* 40.11 (2014): 754.

5. In his book *Reasons and Persons* (Oxford: Clarendon Press, 1984), Derek Parfit began the discussion of the cases in which one must choose whether to create a person who either exists in a handicapped state or does not exist at all, which gave rise to a vast literature about the nonidentity problem.

6. Ronald M. Green, *The Human Embryo Research Debates: Bioethics in the Vortex of Controversy* (Oxford: Oxford University Press, 2001), 126–27.

7. Anna Smajdor and Daniela Cutas, "Artificial Gametes and the Ethics of Unwitting Parenthood," *Journal of Medical Ethics* 40.11 (November 2014): 748–51.

8. Ibid., 749.

9. Smajdor and Cutas, "Artificial Gametes," 750.

10. Judith Jarvis Thomson, "A Defense of Abortion," *Philosophy and Public Affairs* 1 (1971): 47–66.

11. Palacios-González, Harris, and Testa, "Multiplex Parenting," 756.

12. Ibid.

Chapter 4.   Is Roe v. Wade *Unquestionably Correct?*

1. Michelle Ye Hee Lee, "Is the United States One of Seven Countries That 'Allow Elective Abortions after 20 Weeks of Pregnancy'?," *Washington Post*, October 9, 2017, https://www.washingtonpost.com/news/fact-checker/wp/2017/10/09 /is-the-united-states-one-of-seven-countries-that-allow-elective-abortions-after -20-weeks-of-pregnancy/?utm_term=.be069c8d50bd\.

2. Erwin Chemerinsky and Michele Goodwin, "Abortion: A Woman's Private Choice," *Texas Law Review* 95 (2017): 1189–1247.

3. Ibid., 1238.

4. Ibid.

5. Ibid., 1201.

6. Ibid., 1228 (internal citations omitted).

7. Patrick Lee and Melissa Moschella, "Embryology and Science Denial," *Public Discourse*, November 8, 2017, www.thepublicdiscourse.com/2017/11 /20449/.

8. Sarah Knapton, "Human Embryos Kept Alive in Lab for Unprecedented 13 Days So Scientists Can Watch Development," *Telegraph*, May 4, 2016, www .telegraph.co.uk/science/2016/05/04/human-embryos-kept-alive-in-lab-for -unprecedented-13-days-so-sci/.

9. Kate Greasley and Christopher Kaczor, *Abortion Rights: For and Against* (New York: Cambridge University Press, 2018), 6.

10. Chemerinsky and Goodwin, "Abortion," 1229.

11. Ibid.

12. Ibid.

13. Ibid.

14. Germain Grisez writes, "Even true contraceptive acts, considered in moral terms, are contralife, since one who chooses to contracept chooses to prevent a new instance of the basic human good of life." *Living a Christian Life*, vol. 2 of *The Way of the Lord Jesus* (New York: Alba House, 1993), chap. 8, summary, http://twotlj.org/G-2-8-S.html.

15. Indeed, Grisez considers it a mistake to conflate contraception and abortion: "A canon concerning contraception, *Si aliquis*, was included in the Church's universal law from the thirteenth century until 1917: 'If anyone for the sake of satisfying sexual desire or with premeditated hatred does something to a man or to a woman, or gives something to drink, so that he cannot generate, or she cannot conceive, or offspring be born, let that person be treated as a homicide.' This canon does not say contraception is homicide; the tradition made no such mistake. Rather, the canon says that those who use contraception commit a sin analogous to homicide." Grisez, *Living a Christian Life*, vol. 2, chap. 8, question E, http://twotlj.org/G-2-8-E.html.

16. *Catechism of the Catholic Church*, 2003, www.vatican.va/archive/ENG 0015/_INDEX.HTM, 2270.

17. Ibid., 2366.

18. Chemerinsky and Goodwin, "Abortion," 1230.

19. Don Marquis, "Why Abortion Is Immoral," *Journal of Philosophy* 86.4 (1989): 183–202; Robert P. George and Christopher Tollefsen, *Embryo: A Defense of Human Life* (New York: Doubleday, 2008); Patrick Lee, *Abortion and Unborn Human Life* (Washington, DC: Catholic University of America Press, 1996); Francis Beckwith, *Defending Life: A Moral and Legal Case against Abortion Choice* (New York: Cambridge University Press, 2007); Christopher Kaczor, *The Ethics of Abortion: Women's Rights, Human Life, and the Question of Justice*, 2nd ed. (New York: Routledge, 2015).

20. Michael Davis, "A Present Like Ours: A Refutation of Marquis's Argument against Abortion and a Sketch of a General Theory of Personhood," *International Journal of Applied Philosophy* 27.1 (Spring 2013): 75–90, doi: 10.5840 /ijap20132718.

21. Ibid., 88.

22. Ibid.

23. Rob Lovering, "The Substance View: A Critique (Part 2)," *Bioethics* 28.7 (September 2014): 378.

24. See, for example, Kaczor, *Ethics of Abortion*; Beckwith, *Defending Life*; George and Tollefsen, *Embryo*; and P. Lee, *Abortion*.

25. Lovering, "Substance View (2)," 381.

26. Ibid.

27. Edward Feser, *Scholastic Metaphysics: A Contemporary Introduction* (Neunkirchen-Seelscheid, Germany: Editiones Scholasticae, 2015), 233.

28. Lovering, "Substance View (2)," 383.

29. Ibid., 378n2.

30. Ibid., 384.

31. Thomas Aquinas, *Summa theologiae* I-II.94.3 ad 2.

32. Germain Grisez offers other reasons against animal cruelty that do not presuppose that animals have equal rights to human beings; see *Living a Christian Life*, chap. 10, question C, http://www.twotlj.org/G-2-10-C.html.

33. Chemerinsky and Goodwin, "Abortion," 1197, 1200, 1211, 1226.

34. Ibid., 1235.

35. Ibid.

36. Ibid., 1234.

37. Michael Tooley, "Abortion and Infanticide," *Philosophy and Public Affairs* 2.1 (1972): 37–65; Peter Singer, *Writings on an Ethical Life* (New York: Ecco Press, 2000) 160–61; Alberto Giubilini and Francesca Minerva, "After-Birth Abortion: Why Should the Baby Live?" *Journal of Medical Ethics* 39.5 (May 2013): 261–63, doi: 10.1136/medethics-2011-100411.

38. To get some sense of the range of debate and lack of consensus on the issue of newborn personhood, see Julian Savulescu and Peter Singer, eds., "Abortion, Infanticide and Allowing Babies to Die, Forty Years On," special issue, *Journal of Medical Ethics* 39.5 (2013), http://jme.bmj.com/content/39/5.

39. Chemerinsky and Goodwin, "Abortion," 1235–36.

40. See, for example, Christopher Kaczor, "Philosophy and Theology: Is Giving Birth More Dangerous Than Aborting?," *National Catholic Bioethics Quarterly* 14.3 (Autumn 2014): 561–66.

Chapter 5.   *What Are Reproductive Rights?*

1. Muireann Quigley, "A Right to Reproduce?" *Bioethics* 24.8 (October 2010): 403–11.

2. Ibid., 404.

3. See Wesley Hohfeld, "The Rights and Wrongs of Abortion: A Reply to Judith Thomson," *Philosophy and Public Affairs* 2.2 (1973): 117–45.

4. See Hugh LaFollette, "Licensing Parents Revisited," *Journal of Applied Philosophy* 27.4 (November 2010): 327–43; and Joyce C. Havstad, "Human Reproductive Cloning: A Conflict of Liberties," *Bioethics* 24.2 (February 2010): 71–77.

5. Quigley, "Right to Reproduce?"

6. Nellie Wieland, "Parental Obligation," *Utilitas* 23.3 (September 2011): 249–67.

7. Ibid., 255.

8. See, for example, Alasdair MacIntyre, *After Virtue: A Study in Moral Philosophy* (Notre Dame, IN: University of Notre Dame Press, 1981), 148–50; Anthony Lisska, *Aquinas's Theory of Natural Law: An Analytic Reconstruction* (Oxford: Oxford University Press, 1996); and Hilary Putnam, *The Collapse of the Fact/Value Dichotomy and Other Essays* (Cambridge, MA: Harvard University Press, 2002).

9. Wieland, "Parental Obligation," 255, emphases in original.

10. Ibid., 257.

11. Ibid., 259.

12. Robert Sparrow, "Orphaned at Conception: The Uncanny Offspring of Embryos," *Bioethics* 26.4 (May 2012): 174.

13. Ibid., 176.

14. Ibid., 177.

15. Mianna Lotz, "Rethinking Procreation: Why It Matters Why We Have Children," *Journal of Applied Philosophy* 28.2 (May 2011): 105–6.

16. Havstad, "Human Reproductive Cloning," 74.

Chapter 6. Is It Better Never to Have Been Born?

1. Dan Thomas, "Better Never to Have Been Born: Christian Ethics, Anti-abortion Politics, and the Pro-life Paradox," *Journal of Religious Ethics* 44.3 (2016): 518–42, doi: 10.1111/jore.12152.

2. Ibid., 522.

3. Ibid.

4. Ibid., 530.

5. Ibid., 535.

6. Ibid.

7. Ibid., 538.

8. Ibid.

9. Augustine, *De peccatorum meritis et remissione* 1.16.21, ed. C. F. Vrba and Josephus Zycha, CSEL 60 (Vindobonae: F. Tempsky; Lipsiae: G. Freytag, 1913), 20f; Augustine, *Sermo* 294.3, PL 38:1337; Augustine, *Contra Iulianum* 5.11.44, PL 44:809. These citations are culled from the discussion of Augustine's views by the International Theological Commission, "The Hope of Salvation for Infants Who Die without Being Baptized," January 19, 2007, www.vatican.va/roman_curia /congregations/cfaith/cti_documents/rc_con_cfaith_doc_20070419_un-baptised -infants_en.html.

10. Thomas Aquinas, *De malo*, q. 5, art. 3, trans. Jean Oesterle as *On Evil* (Notre Dame, IN: University of Notre Dame Press, 1995).

11. *Catechism of the Catholic Church*, #1261 (2003), www.vatican.va/archive /ENG0015/_INDEX.HTM.

12. Congregation for the Doctrine of the Faith, "Pastoralis actio," n13, *Acta Apostolicae Sedis* 72 (1980): 1144; International Theological Commission, "Hope of Salvation."

13. Christopher Kaczor, *Thomas Aquinas on Faith, Hope, and Love* (Naples, FL: Sapientia Press of Ave Maria University, 2008), 119–23.

14. Avery Dulles, "The Population of Hell," *First Things*, May 2003, https: //www.firstthings.com/.

15. Thomas Aquinas, *Summa theologiae* (hereafter *ST*) III, q. 68, art. 2, ad. 3; all citations are to the translation of Fathers of the English Dominican Province (Notre Dame, IN: Christian Classics, 1947).

16. *ST* III, q. 68, art. 10.

17. *ST* III, q. 68, art. 11, obj. 3.

18. *ST* III, q. 68, art. 11, ad. 3.

19. Thomas Aquinas, *In duo praecepta caritatis et in decem legis praecepta. De dilectione Dei*, vol. 2, para. 1168 of *Opuscula theologica*, ed. Taurinen (1954), 250, quoted in John Paul II, *Veritatis splendor*, sec. 78 (Vatican City: Libreria Editrice Vaticana, 1993).

20. John Paul II, *Veritatis splendor* (Vatican City: Libreria Editrice Vaticana, 1993), sec. 81.

21. John Paul II, *Evangelium vitae* (Vatican City: Liberia Editrice Vaticana, 1995), sec. 62.

22. Ibid.

Chapter 7.   Is There a Right to the Death of the Fetus?

1. A summary of this discussion is found in Christopher Kaczor, *The Ethics of Abortion: Women's Rights, Human Life, and the Question of Justice*, 2nd ed. (New York: Routledge, 2015), chap. 12.

2. Joona Räsänen, "Ectogenesis, Abortion and a Right to the Death of the Fetus," *Bioethics* 31 (2017): 697–702.

3. Ibid., 698.

4. Ibid.

5. See, for example, the appendix of Kaczor, *Ethics of Abortion*.

6. David M. Fergusson, Lynne Horwood, and Elizabeth M. Ridder, "Abortion in Young Women and Subsequent Mental Health," *Journal of Child Psychology and Psychiatry* 47 (2006): 16–24; David M. Fergusson, Lynne Horwood,

and Joseph M. Boden, "Abortion and Mental Health Disorders: Evidence from a 30-Year Longitudinal Study," *British Journal of Psychiatry* 193 (2008): 444–51; David M. Fergusson, Lynne Horwood, and Joseph M. Boden, "Reactions to Abortion and Subsequent Mental Health," *British Journal of Psychiatry* 195 (2009): 420–26.

7. David M. Fergusson, "Abortion Increases Mental Health Risk: Study," interview by Tom Iggulden, *AM*, January 3, 2006, ABC, www.abc.net.au/am /content/2006/s1540914.htm.

8. Fergusson, Horwood, and Boden, "Abortion and Mental Health Disorders," 449, emphasis added.

9. Räsänen, "Ectogenesis, Abortion," 698n11.

10. Ibid., 697.

11. For further reflections on the responsibilities of parents to their offspring, see Bernard Prusak, *Parental Obligations and Bioethics: The Duties of a Creator* (New York: Routledge, 2013).

12. Räsänen, "Ectogenesis, Abortion," 699.

13. Ibid.

14. Ibid., 698n11.

15. Ibid., 699.

16. For more on these fallacies, see Peter Kreeft, *Socratic Logic*, 2nd ed. (South Bend, IN: St. Augustine's Press, 2005), 243–50.

17. Räsänen, "Ectogenesis, Abortion," 702.

18. Ibid., 701.

19. Ibid., 699.

20. Ibid., 700.

21. There are, of course, other arguments that, if correct, would secure the right of parents to secure the death of their fetus. For example, if the arguments given by Alberto Giubilini and Francesca Minerva are right, then parents have the right to kill not only their fetus but also their newborn. See Alberto Giubilini and Francesca Minerva, "After-birth Abortion: Why Should the Baby Live?," *Journal of Medical Ethics* 39.5 (2013): 261–63. For an argument that parents do not have the right to kill their fetus or their newborn, see Kaczor, *Ethics of Abortion*.

Chapter 8.   *Why Should the Baby Live?*

1. Alberto Giubilini and Francesca Minerva, "After-birth Abortion: Why Should the Baby Live?," *Journal of Medical Ethics* 39.5 (2013): 261–63.

2. Ibid., 262n1.

3. Michael Tooley, "Abortion and Infanticide," *Philosophy and Public Affairs* 2.1 (1972): 37–65.

4. Bertha Alvarez Manninen, "Yes, the Baby Should Live: A Pro-choice Response to Giubilini and Minerva," *Journal of Medical Ethics* 39.5 (May 2013): 330–35.

5. John Locke quoted in ibid., 333.

6. Ibid.

7. John Finnis, "Capacity, Harm and Experience in the Life of Persons as Equals," *Journal of Medical Ethics* 39.5 (May 2013): 283.

8. Manninen, "Yes, the Baby Should Live," 333.

9. Ibid., 334, note ii.

10. Jessica Jerreat, "Mother-of-Three Training for a Half Marathon Leaves Practice with a Sore Back, Discovers It's Actually Labor Pains and Gives Birth to a Surprise Baby," *Daily Mail*, June 5, 2013.

11. Neil Levy, "The Moral Significance of Being Born," *Journal of Medical Ethics* 39.5 (May 2013): 327.

12. Regina A. Rini, "Of Course the Baby Should Live: Against 'After-birth Abortion,'" *Journal of Medical Ethics* 39.5 (May 2013): 356.

13. Janelle Weaver, "Social before Birth: Twins First Interact with Each Other as Fetuses: Twins Interact Purposefully in the Womb," *Scientific American*, January 1, 2011.

14. Lindsey Porter, "Abortion, Infanticide and Moral Context," *Journal of Medical Ethics* 39.5 (May 2013): 352.

15. Christopher Kaczor, *The Ethics of Abortion*, 2nd ed. (New York: Routledge, 2015), 17–20.

16. Joona Räsänen, "Pro-life Arguments against Infanticide and Why They Are Not Convincing," *Bioethics* 30 (2016): 656–62.

17. Ibid., 657n4.

18. Judith Jarvis Thomson, "A Defense of Abortion," *Philosophy and Public Affairs* 1 (1971): 47–66.

19. John Finnis, *Moral Absolutes: Tradition, Revision, and Truth* (Washington, DC: Catholic University of America Press, 1991), 78–81.

20. Jeff McMahan, "Killing Embryos for Stem Cell Research," *Metaphilosophy* 38 (2007): 170–89, esp. 177–81.

21. Patrick Lee and Robert P. George, 2008. *Body-Self Dualism in Contemporary Ethics and Policy* (Cambridge: Cambridge University Press, 2008).

22. Kaczor, *Ethics of Abortion*, 92n3, 96–99, 146, 219.

23. Ibid., 96–99n3.

24. Ibid., 92n3, 146, 219.

25. Räsänen, "Pro-life Arguments," 658n4.

26. Ibid., 658.

27. Kaczor, *Ethics of Abortion*, 146n3.

28. Räsänen, "Pro-life Arguments," 658.

29. Räsänen, "Pro-life Arguments," 660n4.

30. Giubilini and Minerva, "After-birth Abortion," 262n1, emphasis in the original.

31. Räsänen, "Pro-life Arguments," 660n4.

Chapter 9.   Do Children Have a Right to Be Loved?

1. Mhairi Cowden, "What's Love Got to Do with It? Why a Child Does Not Have a Right to Be Loved," *Critical Review of International Social and Political Philosophy* 15.3 (June 2011): 325–45.

2. Barbara L. Fredrickson, *Love 2.0: How Our Supreme Emotion Affects Everything We Feel, Think, Do, and Become* (New York: Hudson Street Press, 2013), 17.

3. S. Matthew Liao, "The Right of Children to Be Loved," *Journal of Political Philosophy* 14.4 (2006): 420–40.

4. S. Matthew Liao, "Why Children Need to Be Loved," *Critical Review of International Social and Political Philosophy* 15.3 (January 2012): 347–58.

5. Alexander Pruss, *One Body: An Essay in Christian Sexual Ethics* (Notre Dame, IN: University of Notre Dame Press, 2012), 8–48.

6. Heleana Theixos and S. B. Jamil, "The Bad Habit of Bearing Children," *International Journal of Feminist Approaches to Bioethics* 7.1 (Spring 2014): 35–45.

7. Peter Singer, "Famine, Affluence, and Morality," *Philosophy and Public Affairs* 1.3 (Spring 1972): 241.

8. Karey Harwood, "Bad Habit or Considered Decision: The Need for a Closer Examination of Prospective Parents' Views," *International Journal of Feminist Approaches to Bioethics* 7.1 (Spring 2014): 50.

9. Michel Accad, "Heterologous Embryo Transfer: Magisterial Answers and Metaphysical Questions," *Linacre Quarterly* 81.1 (February 2014): 38–46.

10. Thomas K. Nelson, "Personhood and Embryo Adoption," *Linacre Quarterly* 79.3 (August 2012): 267.

11. Ibid.

12. Ibid., 269.

Chapter 10.   Do Children Contribute to the Flourishing of Their Parents?

1. Germain Grisez and Russell Shaw, *Personal Vocation: God Calls Everyone by Name* (Huntington, IN: Our Sunday Visitor, 2003).

2. John Henry Newman, *Prayers, Verses, and Devotions* (San Francisco: Ignatius Press, 2002), 338.

3. Augustine, *Homilies on the Gospel of St John* 7.8.

4. Thomas Aquinas, *Summa theologiae* (hereafter *ST*) I-II, q. 1–5.

5. George E. Vaillant, *Triumphs of Experience: The Men of the Harvard Grant Study* (Cambridge, MA: Harvard University Press, 2015), 52.

6. Martin Seligman, *Flourish: A Visionary New Understanding of Happiness and Well-Being* (New York: Free Press, 2011), 20.

7. Sigmund Freud, *Civilization and Its Discontents*, trans. James Strachey (New York: W. W. Norton, 1989), 33.

8. C. S. Lewis, *The Four Loves* (New York: Houghton Mifflin Harcourt, 1991), 121.

9. Dan Ariely, *The Upside of Irrationality: The Unexpected Benefits of Defying Logic at Work and at Home* (New York: Harper Perennial, 2011), 83.

10. Alexander Pruss, *One Body: An Essay in Christian Sexual Ethics* (Notre Dame, IN: University of Notre Dame Press, 2012), chap. 2.

11. Jean Vanier, *From Brokenness to Community* (New York: Paulist Press, 1992), 16.

12. Alexander Solzhenitsyn, *The Gulag Archipelago*, trans. Thomas P. Whitney and Harry Willets (New York: Harper Perennial Modern Classics, 2007), 312.

13. *ST* I-II, q. 94, art. 2.

14. William Shakespeare, sonnet 18, lines 7–8.

15. J. R. R. Tolkien, *The Letters of J. R. R. Tolkien*, ed. Humphrey Carpenter (New York: Houghton Mifflin Harcourt, 2014), 51.

16. Bradford W. Wilcox, *Why Marriage Matters: Thirty Conclusions from the Social Sciences*, 3rd ed. (New York: Broadway Publications, 2011).

17. Alex Witchel, "Father Rabbit," *New York Times*, November 22, 1992, www.nytimes.com/1992/11/22/style/father-rabbit.html?pagewanted=all.

18. Second Vatican Council, *Gaudium et spes* (Vatican City: Libreria Editrice Vaticana, 1965), §50.

19. An earlier, less developed articulation of these views is found in Christopher Kaczor, *The Seven Big Myths about Marriage* (San Francisco: Ignatius Press, 2014).

20. I should add a word about people who become parents via adoption. Although they do not have a bond of DNA with their child, people who become parents via adoption are *truly* parents. A couple who adopts a child may say in truth, "This child is ours and ours alone."

21. John Gottman, *The Seven Principles of Making Marriage Work* (New York: Random House, 2015), 19.

22. David Bess, *The Evolution of Desire* (New York: Basic Books, 2003), 175.

23. Of course, raising children does not automatically make a person virtuous. To become virtuous requires a difficult task but not one that completely overwhelms. For this reason, the church encourages "responsible parenthood" rather than maximal reproduction. Responsible parenthood involves practical wisdom about the strengths and weaknesses of the couple, their economic situation, and all the relevant circumstances. To have children contrary to what practical wisdom would warrant is conducive not to virtue but to vice. In a similar way, people are called to be generous to the poor in giving donations, but it would, for most people, be contrary to practical wisdom to give away 90 percent of the family's income. So too, married couples are called to be generous in giving life, but it may be contrary to practical wisdom to have as many children as biologically possible.

24. I do not mean to imply that heaven is an extrinsic reward essentially unrelated to one's earthly life. Heaven and hell, loving God and neighbor or not loving God and neighbor, begins here on earth. The state of being alienated from God here and now comes to its ultimate conclusion at death in the state of continuing to be alienated from God for all eternity. So also, loving God and neighbor in this life can continue and be brought to perfection after death in what we call heaven.

25. This definition of responsible parenthood is from Paul VI, *Humanae vitae*, July 26, 1968, #10, http://w2.vatican.va/content/paul-vi/en/encyclicals/documents/hf_p-vi_enc_25071968_humanae-vitae.html.

26. John Henry Newman, *Parochial and Plain Sermons* (San Francisco: Ignatius Press, 1987), 917.

27. I should add that good parents may, with great regret, come to the conclusion that physical contact with a violent mentally ill child is no longer possible. This lack of physical contact is compatible with unconditional love. Such sad cases are similar to situations in which a spouse may and should separate from a violent or mentally ill spouse. The marital or parental love remains but is sadly imperfect.

28. Elisha Wiesel, "Lessons from My Father: Elie Wiesel's Son on His Rebellion, and His Father's Love," *New York Jewish Week*, June 7, 2017, http://jewishweek.timesofisrael.com/lessons-from-my-father.

29. Before becoming Pope Benedict XVI, Joseph Cardinal Ratzinger had this to say about the meaning of religious celibacy: "The renunciation of marriage and family is thus to be understood in terms of this vision: I renounce what, humanly speaking, is not only the most normal but also the most important thing. I forgo bringing forth further life on the tree of life, and I live in the faith that my land is really God—and so I make it easier for others, also, to believe that there is a kingdom of heaven. I bear witness to Jesus Christ, to the gospel, not only with words, but also with a specific mode of existence, and I place my life in this form at his disposal. . . . The point is really an existence that stakes everything on God and

leaves out precisely the one thing that normally makes a human existence fulfilled with a promising future." Joseph Ratzinger, *Salt of the Earth: Christianity and the Catholic Church at the End of the Millennium: An Interview with Peter Seewald* (San Francisco: Ignatius Press, 1997), 195.

30. United States Supreme Court, Planned Parenthood of Southeastern Pa. v. Casey, 505 U.S. 833, 851 (1992).

31. Jean-Paul Sartre, *Existentialism and Human Emotion* (New York: Castle, 1957), 60.

32. Michael Sandel, *The Case against Perfection: Ethics in the Age of Genetic Engineering* (Cambridge, MA: Belknap Press, 2009).

33. Ralph McInerny, *Aquinas and Analogy* (Washington, DC: Catholic University of America Press, 1998).

34. I should add that fulfilling parental duties does not exhaust the call of Matthew 25. If I am a good father but do not reach out to those outside my family in need whom I can help, I have not fulfilled this commandment. Indeed, part of being good parents is to teach one's children that the circle of love is not limited to family and friends. There is no better way to teach this lesson than by showing them by example and drawing them into the practice of caring for those in need outside the family. For many people, caring deeply for one's own child can loosen the grip of selfishness and open the door to seeing others in need as worthy of care.

Chapter 11.   Is "Death with Dignity" a Dangerous Euphemism?

This chapter is coauthored by Robert P. George.

1. For a more in-depth explanation of the first three senses of the term, see Daniel P. Sulmasy, "Dignity and Bioethics: History, Theory, and Selected Applications," in *Human Dignity and Bioethics: Essays Commissioned by the President's Council on Bioethics*, ed. Edmund D. Pellegrino, Adam Schulman, and Thomas W. Merrill (Washington, DC: US Independent Agencies and Commissions, 2008), 469–501. The fourth sense of the term is suggested by Ruth Macklin, who holds that dignity can be reduced to respect for autonomy. See her article "Dignity Is a Useless Concept," *British Medical Journal* 327.7429 (2003): 1419–20.

2. Sulmasy, "Dignity and Bioethics," 473.

3. Ibid.

4. Ibid.

5. Macklin, "Dignity," 1419, 1420.

6. Perhaps the most well-known defense of Macklin's claim is Steven Pinker's "The Stupidity of Dignity: Conservative Bioethics' Latest, Most Dangerous Ploy," *New Republic*, May 28, 2008. A critique of their views can be found in the

first chapter of Christopher Kaczor's *A Defense of Dignity: Creating Life, Destroying Life, and Protecting the Rights of Conscience*, Notre Dame Studies in Medical Ethics (Notre Dame, IN: University of Notre Dame Press, 2013).

7. See Patrick Lee and Robert P. George, *Body-Self Dualism in Contemporary Ethics and Politics* (New York: Cambridge University Press, 2007).

8. Immanuel Kant, *Grounding for the Metaphysics of Morals*, trans. James W. Ellington, 3rd ed. (Indianapolis: Hackett, 1993), 36.

9. For more on this distinction, see John Keown, *The Law and Ethics of Medicine: Essays on the Inviolability of Human Life* (New York: Oxford University Press, 2012), chap. 1.

10. For more on body-self dualism, see P. Lee and George, *Body-Self Dualism*.

11. Kant, *Grounding*, 35.

12. Ibid., 36.

13. Ibid., 37.

14. Ronald Dworkin et al., "Assisted Suicide: The Philosophers' Brief," *New York Review of Books*, March 27, 1997.

15. Colin Bird, "Dignity as a Moral Concept," *Social Philosophy and Policy* 30.1–2 (January 2013): 150–76.

16. Alan Gewirth, *Self-Fulfillment* (Princeton, NJ: Princeton University Press, 2009), 168–69.

17. Ibid., 169.

18. John Keown, "A New Father for Law and Ethics of Medicine," in *Reason, Morality, and Law: The Philosophy of John Finnis*, ed. John Keown and Robert P. George (Oxford: Oxford University Press, 2013), 300.

19. John Finnis, *Human Rights and Common Good*, vol. 3 of *Collected Essays of John Finnis* (Oxford: Oxford University Press, 2011), 226.

Chapter 12.   Should Euthanasia Be Permitted for Children?

1. Richard John Neuhaus, "The Return of Eugenics," *Commentary Magazine*, April 1, 1988, 19.

2. Luc Bovens, "Child Euthanasia: Should We Just Not Talk about It?," *Journal of Medical Ethics* 41.8 (2015) 630–34, doi: 10.1136/medethics-2014-102329.

3. Ibid., 631.

4. Ibid.

5. Ibid.

6. Ibid., 632.

7. Ann Goldman, "ABC of Palliative Care: Special Problems of Children," *British Medical Journal* 316.7124 (January 3, 1998): 49–52.

8. Bovens, "Child Euthanasia," 632.

9. Udo Schuklenk and Suzanne van de Vathorst, "Treatment-Resistant Major Depressive Disorder and Assisted Dying," *Journal of Medical Ethics* 41.8 (2015): 577, doi: 0.1136/medethics-2014-102458, emphasis in original.

10. Ibid., 578.

11. Ibid., 582.

12. John Keown, *The Law and Ethics of Medicine: Essays on the Inviolability of Human Life* (Oxford: Oxford University Press, 2012). Rather than engage his arguments, Schuklenk and van de Vathorst patronizingly refer to Keown, who holds three doctorates and an endowed chair at Georgetown University, as an "antieuthanasia campaigner."

13. See Immanuel Kant, *Grounding for the Metaphysics of Morals*, trans. James E. Ellington (Indianapolis: Hackett, 1993), 70.

14. Thomas Aquinas, *Summa theologiae* II-II, q. 64, art. 5, trans. Fathers of the English Dominican Province (Notre Dame, IN: Christian Classics, 1947).

15. Schuklenk and van de Vathorst, "Treatment-Resistant Major Depressive Disorder," 579.

16. See Neuhaus, "Return of Eugenics," 19.

Chapter 13.   Does Assisted Suicide Harm Those Who Do Not Choose to Die?

This chapter was written with the help of Robert Spitzer, S.J.

1. Barry Schwartz, *The Paradox of Choice: Why More Is Less* (New York: HarperCollins, 2004).

2. Hal Bernton, "Washington's Initiative 1000 Is Modeled on Oregon's Death with Dignity Act," *Seattle Times,* October 13, 2008.

3. Madelyn Gould, Patrick Jamieson, and Daniel Romer, "Media Contagion and Suicide among the Young," *American Behavioral Scientist* 46.9 (2003) 1269–84, doi: 10.1177/0002764202250670.

Chapter 14.   Is Conscientious Objection to Abortion Like Conscientious Objection to Antibiotics?

1. Alberto Giubilini and Francesca Minerva, "After-birth Abortion: Why Should the Baby Live?," *Journal of Medical Ethics* 39.5 (May 2013): 261–63, doi: 10.1136/medethics-2011-100411.

2. Alberto Giubilini, "Objection to Conscience: An Argument against Conscience Exemptions in Healthcare," *Bioethics* 31.5 (June 2017): 400, doi:10.1111 /bioe.12333.

3. Ibid., 404.

4. Ibid., 408.

5. Ibid., 404.

6. On vitalism, the inviolability of life, and the quality of life, see John Keown, *The Law and Ethics of Medicine: Essays on the Inviolability of Human Life* (Oxford: Oxford University Press, 2012).

7. Giubilini, "Objection to Conscience," 404.

8. On the question of the safety of abortion, see Christopher Kaczor, *The Ethics of Abortion: Women's Rights, Human Life, and the Question of Justice*, 2nd ed. (Routledge: New York, 2015). See too David M. Fergusson, Lynne Horwood, and Joseph M. Boden, "Abortion and Mental Health Disorders: Evidence from a 30-Year Longitudinal Study," *British Journal of Psychiatry* 193 (2008): 449, emphasis added.

9. Giubilini and Minerva, "After-birth Abortion," 263.

10. F. Parazzini et al., "Induced Abortions and Risk of Ectopic Pregnancy," *Human Reproduction* 10.7 (July 1995): 1841–44; Jyotindu Debnath et al., "Ectopic Pregnancy in the Era of Medical Abortion: Are We Ready for It? Spectrum of Sonographic Findings and Our Experience in a Tertiary Care Service Hospital of India," *Journal of Obstetrics and Gynecology of India* 63.6 (November–December 2013): 388–93, doi: 10.1007/s13224-013-0459-2; and Osaheni L. Lawani, Okechukwu B. Anozie, and Paul O. Ezeonu, "Ectopic Pregnancy: A Life-Threatening Gynecological Emergency," *International Journal of Women's Health* 5 (July 15, 2013): 515–21, doi: 10.2147/IJWH.S49672.

11. Giubilini, "Objection to Conscience," 404.

12. Nancy Berlinger, "Conscience Clauses, Healthcare Providers, and Parents," in *From Birth to Death and Bench to Clinic: The Hastings Center Bioethics Briefing Book for Journalists, Policymakers, and Campaigns*, ed. Mary Crowley (Garrison, NY: Hastings Center, 2008), 35.

13. Giubilini, "Objection to Conscience," 405.

14. Ibid.

15. See Gerard V. Bradley, "The Future of Pro-life Legislation and Litigation," *Public Discourse*, October 18, 2016, www.thepublicdiscourse.com/.

16. Giubilini, "Objection to Conscience," 406.

17. Alvin Plantinga, *Where the Conflict Really Lies: Science, Religion, and Naturalism* (Oxford: Oxford University Press, 2011).

18. Donald Marquis, "Why Abortion Is Immoral," *Journal of Philosophy* 86.4 (April 1989): 183–202. See also Don Marquis, "Abortion Revisited," in *The Oxford Handbook of Bioethics*, ed. Bonnie Steinbock (Oxford: Oxford University Press, 2007), 395–415.

19. See Kaczor, *Ethics of Abortion*; Robert P. George and Christopher Tollefsen, *Embryo: A Defense of Human Life* (New York: Doubleday, 2008);

and Patrick Lee, *Abortion and Unborn Human Life*, 2nd ed. (Washington, DC: Catholic University of America Press, 2010).

20. Giubilini and Minerva, "After-birth Abortion," 263.

Chapter 15.   Do Medical Conscientious Objectors Differ from Military Conscientious Objectors?

1. R. Y. Stahl and E. J. Emanuel, "Physicians, Not Conscripts: Conscientious Objection in Health Care," *New England Journal of Medicine* 376.14 (2017): 1380–85, doi: 10.1056/NEJMsb1612472.

2. Ibid., 1383.

3. Ibid., 1381.

4. Ibid.

5. US Conference of Catholic Bishops, *The Catholic Church in America: Meeting Real Needs in Your Neighborhood* (Washington, DC: Catholic Information Project, 2006), 12.

6. Stahl and Emanuel, "Physicians, Not Conscripts," 1381.

7. Ibid.

8. Ibid., 1382.

9. Ibid., 1381.

10. Ibid.

11. Ibid.

12. Ibid., 1382.

13. Plato, *Gorgias*, 508e–509d, trans. Walter Hamilton (New York: Penguin Books, 1960): "Any wrong whatsoever done to me or mine, are both worse and more shameful to the wrongdoer than to me the wronged."

14. See, for example, Christopher Kaczor, *A Defense of Dignity: Creating Life, Destroying Life, and Protecting the Rights of Conscience*, Notre Dame Studies in Medical Ethics (Notre Dame, IN: University of Notre Dame Press, 2013), chaps. 12 and 13.

Chapter 16.   Should Conscientiously Objecting Institutions Cover Elective Abortion in Their Insurance Plans?

1. Ian Lovett, "Abortion Vote Exposes Rift at a Catholic University," *New York Times*, October 6, 2013, www.nytimes.com/2013/10/07/us/abortion-vote-exposes-rift-at-catholic-university.html?_r=0.

2. "Mixed Messages," *Angelus News*, October 16, 2013, https://angelusnews
.com/news/mixed-messages.

3. Ibid.

4. Roberto Dell'Oro, "Only One Message: LMU Remains Catholic,"
Tidings, October 30, 2013.

5. Ibid.

6. Ibid.

7. Ibid.

8. Ibid.

9. Aristotle, *Nicomachean Ethics* 1107a12, trans. Terrence Irwin, 2nd ed. (Indianapolis: Hackett, 1999).

10. Dell'Oro, "Only One Message."

11. Ibid.

12. Provincials of the Society of Jesus in the United States, *Standing for
the Unborn: A Statement of the Society of Jesus in the United States on Abortion*,
March 25, 2003, www.jesuit.org/jesuits/wp-content/uploads/standing-for-the
-unborn.pdf.

Chapter 17.   *Is It Ethically Permissible to Separate Conjoined Twins?*

1. Krzysztof Kobylarz, "History of Treatment of Conjoined Twins," *Anaesthesiology Intensive Therapy* 46 (2014): 116–23.

2. Ibid., 122.

3. John Finnis, "The Other F-Word," *Public Discourse*, October 20, 2010,
www.thepublicdiscourse.com/2010/10/1849/.

4. As cited by Irven Michael Resnick, "Conjoined Twins, Medieval Biology,
and Evolving Reflection on Individual Identity," *Viator* 44 (2013): 344.

5. Ibid., 362.

6. Ibid., 363.

7. Ibid.

8. This medieval debate finds an analogue in contemporary discussions of
human identity and individuality. For example, Eric Olson examines questions
such as whether conjoined twins are two organisms but only one person. See
Eric T. Olson, "The Metaphysical Implications of Conjoined Twinning," *Southern Journal of Philosophy* 52.S1 (2014): 24–40.

9. M. A. Lee, A. K. Gosain, and D. Becker, "The Bioethics of Separating
Conjoined Twins in Plastic Surgery," *Plastic Reconstructive Surgery* 128 (2011):
328e–334e.

10. John Finnis, Germain Grisez, and Joseph Boyle, "'Direct' and 'Indirect':
A Reply to Critics of Our Action Theory," *Thomist* 65 (2001): 1–44.

11. Stephen Brock, "*Veritatis Splendor* §78, St. Thomas, and (Not Merely) Physical Objects of Moral Acts," *Nova et Vetera* (English ed.) 6.1 (2008): 1–62; Lawrence Dewan, "St. Thomas, Rhonheimer, and the Object of the Human Act," *Nova et Vetera* (English ed.) 6.1 (2008): 63–112; Kevin Flannery, "Aristotle and Human Movements," *Nova et Vetera* (English ed.) 6.1 (2008): 113–38.

12. Matthew B. O'Brien and Robert C. Koons, "Objects of Intention: A Hylomorphic Critique of the New Natural Law Theory," *American Catholic Philosophical Quarterly* 86.4 (2012): 656.

13. Ibid., 687–88.

14. Christopher Kaczor, "Intention, Foresight, and Mutilation: A Response to Giebel," *International Philosophical Quarterly* 47 (2007): 478n2.

15. M. Cathleen Kaveny, "The Case of Conjoined Twins: Embodiment, Individuality, and Dependence," *Theological Studies* 62 (2001): 760.

16. Ibid., 776.

17. Ibid.

18. Ibid., 777.

19. Ibid.

20. Ibid., 772.

21. Daniel Gilbert, *Stumbling on Happiness* (New York: Vintage Books, 2006), 32.

22. Ibid.

23. Resnick, "Conjoined Twins," 354.

24. M. Cathleen Kaveny, "Virtuous Decision-Makers and Incompetent Patients: The Case of the Conjoined Twins," In *A Just and True Love: Feminism at the Frontiers of Theological Ethics*, ed. Maura A. Ryan and Brian F. Linnane (Notre Dame, IN: University of Notre Dame Press), 349.

25. Ibid., 335.

Bibliography

Accad, Michel. "Heterologous Embryo Transfer: Magisterial Answers and Meta-physical Questions." *Linacre Quarterly* 81.1 (2014): 38–46.

Anscombe, G. E. M. *Human Life, Action and Ethics: Essays by G. E. M. Anscombe.* St Andrews Studies in Philosophy and Public Affairs. Edited by John Haldane. Exeter: Imprint Academic, 2006.

Aquinas, Thomas. *De malo.* Translated by Jean Oesterle as *On Evil.* Notre Dame, IN: University of Notre Dame Press, 1995.

———. *In duo praecepta caritatis et in decem legis praecepta.* In *De dilectione Dei,* vol. 2 of *Opuscula theologica.* Edited by Taurinen, 1954.

———. *Sententia libri Politicorum.* Translated by Ernest L. Fortin and Peter D. O'Neill as *Commentary on Aristotle's "Politics."* New York: Free Press of Glencoe, 1963. Book 1, lesson 1 available at https://dhspriory.org/thomas/Politics.htm.

———. *Summa contra gentiles, Book 3.* Edited and translated by Vernon J. Bourke. Notre Dame, IN: University of Notre Dame Press, 1975.

———. *Summa theologiae.* Translated by Fathers of the English Dominican Province. Notre Dame, IN: Christian Classics, 1947.

Ariely, Dan. *The Upside of Irrationality: The Unexpected Benefits of Defying Logic at Work and at Home.* New York: Harper, 2010.

Aristotle. *Nicomachean Ethics.* Translated by Terrence Irwin. 2nd ed. Indianapolis: Hackett, 1999.

Augustine. *Contra Iulianum.* PL 44.

———. *De peccatorum meritis et remissione.* Edited by C. F. Vrba and Josephus Zycha. CSEL 60. Vindobonae: F. Tempsky; Lipsiae: G. Freytag, 1913.

———. *Homilies on the Gospel of St. John.* Veritatis Splendor Publications [online platform], 2012.

———. *Sermones.* PL 38.

Australian Broadcasting Corporation. "AM Radio Transcript: Abortion Increases Mental Health Risk." *AM*, October 23, 2017. https://www.abc.net.au/am /content/2006/s1540914.htm.

Baumeister, Roy F., Kathleen D. Vohs, Jennifer Aaker, and Emily N. Garbinsky. "Some Key Differences between a Happy Life and a Meaningful Life." *Journal of Positive Psychology* 8.6 (2013): 505–16.

Beckwith, Francis. "Defending Abortion Philosophically: A Review of David Boonin's *A Defense of Abortion.*" *Journal of Medicine and Philosophy* 31 (2006): 177–203.

————. *Defending Life: A Moral and Legal Case against Abortion Choice*. New York: Cambridge University Press, 2007.

Berlinger, Nancy. "Conscience Clauses, Healthcare Providers, and Parents." In *From Birth to Death and Bench to Clinic: The Hastings Center Bioethics Briefing Book for Journalists, Policymakers, and Campaigns*, edited by Mary Crowley, 35–40. Garrison, NY: Hastings Center, 2008.

Bernton, Hal. "Washington's Initiative 1000 Is Modeled on Oregon's Death with Dignity Act." *Seattle Times*, October 13, 2008.

Bess, David. *The Evolution of Desire*. New York: Basic Books, 2003.

Bird, Colin. "Dignity as a Moral Concept." *Social Philosophy and Policy* 30.1–2 (2013): 150–76.

Boden, Joseph M., David M. Fergusson, and John L. Horwood. "Experience of Sexual Abuse in Childhood and Abortion in Adolescence and Early Adulthood." *Child Abuse and Neglect* 33.12 (2009): 870–76.

Bovens, Luc. "Child Euthanasia: Should We Just Not Talk about It?" *Journal of Medical Ethics* 41.8 (2015): 630–34.

Bradley, Gerard V. "The Future of Pro-life Legislation and Litigation." *Public Discourse*, October 18, 2016.

Brock, Stephen. "*Veritatis Splendor* §78, St. Thomas, and (Not Merely) Physical Objects of Moral Acts." *Nova et Vetera* (English ed.) 6.1 (2008): 1–62.

Catechism of the Catholic Church. 2003. www.vatican.va/archive/ENG0015 /_INDEX.HTM.

Chemerinsky, Erwin, and Michelle Goodwin. "Abortion: A Woman's Private Choice." *Texas Law Review* 95 (2017): 1189–247.

Congregation for the Doctrine of the Faith. "Pastoralis actio." *Acta Apostolicae Sedis* 72 (1980): 1144.

Cowden, Mhairi. "What's Love Got to Do with It? Why a Child Does Not Have a Right to Be Loved." *Critical Review of International Social and Political Philosophy* 15.3 (2011): 325–45.

Craddock, Joshua J. "Protecting Prenatal Persons: Does the Fourteenth Amendment Prohibit Abortion?" *Harvard Journal of Law and Public Policy* 40.2 (2017): 539–72.

Cutas, Daniela, Wybo Dondorp, Tsjalling Swierstra, Sjoerd Repping, and Guido de Wert. "Artificial Gametes: Perspectives of Geneticists, Ethicists, and Representatives of Potential Users." *Medicine, Health Care, and Philosophy* 17.3 (2014): 339–45.

Davis, Michael. "A Present Like Ours: A Refutation of Marquis's Argument against Abortion and a Sketch of a General Theory of Personhood." *International Journal of Applied Philosophy* 27.1 (2013): 75–90. doi: 10.5840/ijap20132718.

Debnath, Jyotindu, Surendra Kumar Gulati, Ankit Mathur, Ritu Gupta, Nikhilesh Kumar, Sunil Arora, and R. Bala Murali Krishna. "Ectopic Pregnancy in the Era of Medical Abortion: Are We Ready for It? Spectrum of Sonographic Findings and Our Experience in a Tertiary Care Service Hospital of India." *Journal of Obstetrics and Gynecology of India* 63.6 (2013): 388–93. doi: 10.1007/s13224-013-0459-2.

DeGrazia, David. "Modal Personhood and Moral Status: A Reply to Kagan's Proposal." *Journal of Applied Philosophy* 33.1 (2016): 22–25.

Dell'Oro, Roberto. "Only One Message: LMU Remains Catholic." *Tidings*, October 30, 2013.

Dewan, Lawrence. "St. Thomas, Rhonheimer, and the Object of the Human Act." *Nova et Vetera* (English ed.) 6.1 (2008): 63–112.

Dulles, Avery. "The Population of Hell." *First Things*, May 2003. https://www.firstthings.com/.

Dworkin, Ronald, Thomas Nagel, Robert Nozick, John Rawls, Judith Jarvis Thomson, et al. "Assisted Suicide: The Philosophers' Brief." *New York Review of Books*, March 27, 1997.

Ebert, Roger. "How I Am a Roman Catholic." *Roger Ebert's Journal*, March 1, 2013. https://www.rogerebert.com/rogers-journal/how-i-am-a-roman-catholic.

Fergusson, David M. "Abortion Increases Mental Health Risk: Study." Interview by Tom Iggulden. *AM*, January 3, 2006, ABC. www.abc.net.au/am/content/2006/s1540914.htm.

Fergusson, David M., Lynne Horwood, and Joseph M. Boden. "Abortion and Mental Health Disorders: Evidence from a 30-Year Longitudinal Study." *British Journal of Psychiatry* 193.6 (2008): 444–51.

———. "Reactions to Abortion and Subsequent Mental Health." *British Journal of Psychiatry* 195.5 (2009): 420–26.

Fergusson, David M., Lynne Horwood, and Elizabeth M. Ridder. "Abortion in Young Women and Subsequent Mental Health." *Journal of Child Psychology and Psychiatry* 47.1 (2006): 16–24.

Feser, Edward. *Scholastic Metaphysics: A Contemporary Introduction*. Neunkirchen-Seelscheid, Germany: Editiones Scholasticae, 2014.

Finnis, John. "Capacity, Harm and Experience in the Life of Persons as Equals." *Journal of Medical Ethics* 39.5 (2013): 281–83.

———. *Human Rights and Common Good.* Vol. 3 of *Collected Essays of John Finnis.* Oxford: Oxford University Press, 2011.

———. *Moral Absolutes: Tradition, Revision, and Truth.* Washington, DC: Catholic University of America Press, 1991.

———. "The Other F-Word." *Public Discourse,* October 20, 2010. www.the publicdiscourse.com/2010/10/1849/.

Finnis, John, Germain Grisez, and Joseph Boyle. "'Direct' and 'Indirect': A Reply to Critics of Our Action Theory." *Thomist* 65.1 (2001): 1–44.

Flannery, Kevin. "Aristotle and Human Movements." *Nova et Vetera* (English ed.) 6.1 (2008): 113–38.

Fredrickson, Barbara L. *Love 2.0: How Our Supreme Emotion Affects Everything We Feel, Think, Do, and Become.* New York: Hudson Street Press, 2013.

Freud, Sigmund. *Civilization and Its Discontents.* New York: W. W. Norton, 1989.

George, Robert P., and Christopher Tollefsen. *Embryo: A Defense of Human Life.* New York: Doubleday, 2008.

Gewirth, Alan. *Self-Fulfillment.* Princeton, NJ: Princeton University Press, 2009.

Gilbert, Daniel. *Stumbling on Happiness.* New York: Vintage Books, 2006.

Girgis, Sherif. "Equality and Moral Worth in Natural Law Ethics and Beyond." *American Journal of Jurisprudence* 59.2 (2014): 143–62.

Giubilini, Alberto. "Objection to Conscience: An Argument against Conscience Exemptions in Healthcare." *Bioethics* 31.5 (2017): 400–408. doi:10.1111/bioe .12333.

Giubilini, Alberto, and Francesca Minerva. "After-birth Abortion: Why Should the Baby Live?" *Journal of Medical Ethics* 39.5 (2013): 261–63. doi: 10.1136 /medethics-2011-100411.

Goldman, Ann. "ABC of Palliative Care: Special Problems of Children." *British Medical Journal* 316.7124 (1998): 49–52.

Gottman, John. *The Seven Principles of Making Marriage Work.* New York: Random House, 2015.

Gould, Madelyn, Patrick Jamieson, and Daniel Romer. "Media Contagion and Suicide among the Young." *American Behavioral Scientist* 46.9 (2003): 1269–84. doi: 10.1177/0002764202250670.

Greasley, Kate, and Christopher Kaczor. *Abortion Rights: For and Against.* New York: Cambridge University Press, 2018.

Green, Ronald. *The Human Embryo Research Debates: Bioethics in the Vortex of Controversy.* Oxford: Oxford University Press, 2001.

Grisez, Germain. *Living a Christian Life.* Vol. 2 of *The Way of the Lord Jesus.* New York: Alba House, 1993. http://twotlj.org.

Grisez, Germain, and Russell Shaw. *Personal Vocation: God Calls Everyone by Name.* Huntington, IN: Our Sunday Visitor, 2003.

Harwood, Karey. "Bad Habit or Considered Decision: The Need for a Closer Examination of Prospective Parents' Views." *International Journal of Feminist Approaches to Bioethics* 7.1 (2014): 46–50.

Havstad, Joyce C. "Human Reproductive Cloning: A Conflict of Liberties." *Bioethics* 24.2 (2010): 71–77.

Hohfeld, Wesley. "The Rights and Wrongs of Abortion: A Reply to Judith Thomson." *Philosophy and Public Affairs* 2.2 (1973): 117–45.

Hughes, Glenn. "The Concept of Dignity in the Universal Declaration of Human Rights." *Journal of Religious Ethics* 39.1 (2011): 1–24.

International Commission on English in the Liturgy. *The Order of Celebrating Matrimony.* 2nd ed. Washington, DC: US Conference of Catholic Bishops, 2016.

International Theological Commission. "The Hope of Salvation for Infants Who Die without Being Baptized." 2007. www.vatican.va/roman_curia /congregations/cfaith/cti_documents/rc_con_cfaith_doc_20070419 _un-baptised-infants_en.html.

Jerreat, Jessica. "Mother-of-Three Training for a Half Marathon Leaves Practice with a Sore Back, Discovers It's Actually Labor Pains and Gives Birth to a Surprise Baby." *Daily Mail,* June 5, 2013.

John Paul II. *Evangelium vitae.* Vatican City: Libreria Editrice Vaticana, 1995.

———. *Veritatis splendor.* Vatican City: Libreria Editrice Vaticana, 1993.

Kaczor, Christopher. *A Defense of Dignity: Creating Life, Destroying Life, and Protecting the Rights of Conscience.* Notre Dame Studies in Medical Ethics. Notre Dame, IN: University of Notre Dame Press, 2013.

———. *The Ethics of Abortion: Women's Rights, Human Life, and the Question of Justice.* 2nd ed. New York: Routledge, 2015.

———. "Intention, Foresight, and Mutilation: A Response to Giebel." *International Philosophical Quarterly* 47 (2007): 477–82.

———. "Philosophy and Theology: Is Giving Birth More Dangerous Than Aborting?" *National Catholic Bioethics Quarterly* 14.3 (2014): 561–66.

———. *The Seven Big Myths about Marriage.* San Francisco: Ignatius Press, 2014.

———. *Thomas Aquinas on Faith, Hope, and Love.* Naples, FL: Sapientia Press of Ave Maria University, 2008.

Kagan, Shelly. "What's Wrong with Speciesism?" Society for Applied Philosophy Annual Lecture 2015. *Journal of Applied Philosophy* 33.1 (2016): 1–21. doi: 10.1111/japp.12164.

Kant, Immanuel. *Grounding for the Metaphysics of Morals.* Translated by James E. Ellington. Indianapolis: Hackett, 1993.

Kaveny, M. Cathleen. "The Case of Conjoined Twins: Embodiment, Individuality, and Dependence." *Theological Studies* 62.4 (2001): 753–86.

————. "Virtuous Decision-Makers and Incompetent Patients: The Case of the Conjoined Twins." In *A Just and True Love: Feminism at the Frontiers of Theological Ethics*, edited by Maura A. Ryan and Brian F. Linnane, 338–68. Notre Dame, IN: University of Notre Dame Press, 2007.

Keown, John. *The Law and Ethics of Medicine: Essays on the Inviolability of Human Life*. New York: Oxford University Press, 2012.

————. "A New Father for Law and Ethics of Medicine." In *Reason, Morality, and Law: The Philosophy of John Finnis*, edited by John Keown and Robert P. George, 290–310. Oxford: Oxford University Press, 2013.

Keown, John, and Robert P. George, eds. *Reason, Morality, and Law: The Philosophy of John Finnis*. Oxford: Oxford University Press, 2013.

Knapton, Sarah. "Human Embryos Kept Alive in Lab for Unprecedented 13 Days So Scientists Can Watch Development." *Telegraph*, May 4, 2016. www .telegraph.co.uk/science/2016/05/04/human-embryos-kept-alive-in-lab-for -unprecedented-13-days-so-sci/.

Kobylarz, Krzysztof. "History of Treatment of Conjoined Twins." *Anaesthesiology Intensive Therapy* 46 (2014): 116–23.

Kreeft, Peter. *Socratic Logic*. 2nd ed. South Bend, IN: St. Augustine's Press, 2005.

LaFollette, Hugh. "Licensing Parents Revisited." *Journal of Applied Philosophy* 27.4 (2010): 327–43.

Lawani, Osaheni L., Okechukwu B. Anozie, and Paul O. Ezeonu. "Ectopic Pregnancy: A Life-Threatening Gynecological Emergency." *International Journal of Women's Health* 5 (2013): 515–21. doi: 10.2147/IJWH.S49672.

Lee, M. A., A. K. Gosain, and D. Becker. "The Bioethics of Separating Conjoined Twins in Plastic Surgery." *Plastic Reconstructive Surgery* 128 (2011): 328e–34e.

Lee, Patrick. *Abortion and Unborn Human Life*. Washington, DC: Catholic University of America Press, 1996.

Lee, Patrick, and Robert P. George. *Body-Self Dualism in Contemporary Ethics and Politics*. New York: Cambridge University Press, 2007.

Lee, Patrick, and Melissa Moschella. "Embryology and Science Denial." *Public Discourse*, November 8, 2017. www.thepublicdiscourse.com/2017/11/20449/.

Leget, Carlo. "Analyzing Dignity: A Perspective from the Ethics of Care." *Medicine, Health Care and Philosophy* 16.4 (2013): 945–52.

Levy, Neil. "The Moral Significance of Being Born." *Journal of Medical Ethics* 39.5 (2013): 326–29.

Lewis, C. S. *The Four Loves*. New York: Houghton Mifflin Harcourt, 1991.

Liao, S. Matthew. "The Right of Children to Be Loved." *Journal of Political Philosophy* 14.4 (2006): 420–40.

————. "Why Children Need to Be Loved." *Critical Review of International Social and Political Philosophy* 15.3 (2012): 347–58.

Lisska, Anthony. *Aquinas's Theory of Natural Law: An Analytic Reconstruction.* Oxford: Oxford University Press, 1996.

Lotz, Mianna. "Rethinking Procreation: Why It Matters Why We Have Children." *Journal of Applied Philosophy* 28.2 (May 2011): 105–21.

Lovering, Rob. "The Substance View: A Critique (Part 2)." *Bioethics* 28.7 (2014): 378–86.

Lovett, Ian. "Abortion Vote Exposes Rift at a Catholic University." *New York Times*, October 6, 2013. www.nytimes.com/2013/10/07/us/abortion-vote-exposes-rift-at-catholic-university.html?_r=0.

MacIntyre, Alasdair. *After Virtue: A Study in Moral Theory.* Notre Dame, IN: University of Notre Dame, 1981.

Macklin, Ruth. "Dignity Is a Useless Concept." *British Medical Journal* 327.7429 (2003): 1419–20.

Manninen, Bertha Alvarez. "Yes, the Baby Should Live: A Pro-choice Response to Giubilini and Minerva." *Journal of Medical Ethics* 39.5 (2013): 330–35.

Marquis, Donald. "Abortion Revisited." In *The Oxford Handbook of Bioethics*, edited by Bonnie Steinbock, 395–415. New York: Oxford University Press, 2007.

———. "Why Abortion Is Immoral." *Journal of Philosophy* 86.4 (1989): 183–202.

McInerny, Ralph. *Aquinas and Analogy.* Washington, DC: Catholic University of America Press, 1998.

McMahan, Jeff. "Killing Embryos for Stem Cell Research." *Metaphilosophy* 38.2–3 (2007): 170–89.

———. "On 'Modal Personism.'" *Journal of Applied Philosophy* 33.1 (2016): 26–30.

"Mixed Messages." *Angelus News*, October 16, 2013. https://angelusnews.com/news/mixed-messages.

Nelson, Thomas K. " Personhood and Embryo Adoption." *Linacre Quarterly* 79.3 (2012): 261–74.

Neuhaus, Richard John. "The Return of Eugenics." *Commentary Magazine* 85.4 (1988): 15–26.

Newman, John Henry. *Parochial and Plain Sermons.* San Francisco: Ignatius Press, 1987.

———. *Prayers, Verses, and Devotions.* San Francisco: Ignatius Press, 2002.

O'Brien, Matthew B., and Robert C. Koons. "Objects of Intention: A Hylomorphic Critique of the New Natural Law Theory." *American Catholic Philosophical Quarterly* 86.4 (2012): 655–703.

Olson, Eric T. "The Metaphysical Implications of Conjoined Twinning." *Southern Journal of Philosophy* 52.S1 (2014): 24–40.

Palacios-González, César, John Harris, and Giuseppe Testa. "Multiplex Parenting: IVG and the Generations to Come." *Journal of Medical Ethics* 40.11 (2014): 752–58.

Parazzini, F., M. Ferraroni, L. Tozzi, E. Ricci, R. Mezzopane, and C. La Vecchia. "Induced Abortions and Risk of Ectopic Pregnancy." *Human Reproduction* 10.7 (1995): 1841–44.

Parfit, Derek. *Reasons and Persons*. New York: Oxford University Press, 1987.

Paul VI. *Humanae vitae*. July 26, 1968. http://w2.vatican.va/content/paul-vi/en/encyclicals/documents/hf_p-vi_enc_25071968_humanae-vitae.html.

Pinker, Steven. "The Stupidity of Dignity: Conservative Bioethics' Latest, Most Dangerous Ploy." *New Republic*, May 28, 2009.

Plantinga, Alvin. *Where the Conflict Really Lies: Science, Religion, and Naturalism*. Oxford: Oxford University Press, 2011.

Plato. *Gorgias*. Translated by Walter Hamilton. New York: Penguin Books, 1971.

Porter, Lindsey. "Abortion, Infanticide and Moral Context." *Journal of Medical Ethics* 39.5 (2013): 350–52.

Provincials of the Society of Jesus in the United States. *Standing for the Unborn: A Statement of the Society of Jesus in the United States on Abortion*. March 25, 2003. www.jesuit.org/jesuits/wp-content/uploads/standing-for-the-unborn.pdf.

Prusak, Bernard. *Parental Obligations and Bioethics: The Duties of a Creator*. New York: Routledge, 2013.

Pruss, Alexander. *One Body: An Essay in Christian Sexual Ethics*. Notre Dame, IN: University of Notre Dame Press, 2012.

Putnam, Hilary. *The Collapse of the Fact/Value Dichotomy and Other Essays*. Cambridge, MA: Harvard University Press, 2002.

Quigley, Muireann. "A Right to Reproduce?" *Bioethics* 24.8 (2010): 403–11.

Ranganathan, Bharat. "Should Inherent Human Dignity Be Considered Intrinsically Heuristic?" *Journal of Religious Ethics* 42.4 (2014): 770–75.

Räsänen, Joona. "Ectogenesis, Abortion and a Right to the Death of the Fetus." *Bioethics* 31.9 (2017): 697–702.

———. "Pro-life Arguments against Infanticide and Why They Are Not Convincing." *Bioethics* 30.9 (2016): 656–62.

Ratzinger, Joseph. *Salt of the Earth: Christianity and the Catholic Church at the End of the Millennium: An Interview with Peter Seewald*. San Francisco: Ignatius Press, 1997.

Resnick, Irven Michael. "Conjoined Twins, Medieval Biology, and Evolving Reflection on Individual Identity." *Viator* 44 (2013): 343–68.

Rini, Regina A. "Of Course the Baby Should Live: Against 'After-birth Abortion.'" *Journal of Medical Ethics* 39.5 (2013): 353–56.

Sandel, Michael. *The Case against Perfection: Ethics in the Age of Genetic Engineering*. Cambridge, MA: Belknap Press, 2009.

Sartre, Jean-Paul. *Existentialism and Human Emotion*. New York City: Castle, 1957.

Savulescu, Julian, and Peter Singer, eds. "Abortion, Infanticide and Allowing Babies to Die, Forty Years On." Special issue, *Journal of Medical Ethics* 39.5 (2013). http://jme.bmj.com/content/39/5.

Schuklenk, Udo, and Suzanne Van de Vathorst. "Treatment-Resistant Major Depressive Disorder and Assisted Dying." *Journal of Medical Ethics* 41.8 (2015): 589–91. doi: 0.1136/medethics-2014-102458.

Schwartz, Barry. *The Paradox of Choice: Why More Is Less*. New York: HarperCollins, 2004.

Second Vatican Council. *Gaudium et spes*. Vatican City: Libreria Editrice Vaticana, 1965.

Seligman, Martin. *Flourish: A Visionary New Understanding of Happiness and Well-Being*. New York: Free Press, 2011.

Singer, Peter. "Famine, Affluence, and Morality." *Philosophy and Public Affairs* 1.3 (Spring 1972): 229–43.

———. "Why Speciesism Is Wrong: A Response to Kagan." *Journal of Applied Philosophy* 33.1 (2016): 31–35. doi: 10.1111/japp.12165.

———. *Writings on an Ethical Life*. New York: Ecco Press, 2000.

Smajdor, Anna, and Daniela Cutas. "Artificial Gametes and the Ethics of Unwitting Parenthood." *Journal of Medical Ethics* 40.11 (November 2014): 748–51.

Solzhenitsyn, Alexander. *The Gulag Archipelago*. Translated by Thomas P. Whitney and Harry Willets. New York: Harper Perennial Modern Classics, 2007.

Sparrow, Robert. "Orphaned at Conception: The Uncanny Offspring of Embryos." *Bioethics* 26.4 (2012): 173–81.

Stahl, Ronit Y., and Ezekiel J. Emanuel. "Physicians, Not Conscripts: Conscientious Objection in Health Care." *New England Journal of Medicine* 376.14 (2017): 1380–85. doi: 10.1056/NEJMsb1612472.

Stossel, Scott. "What Makes Us Happy, Revisited." *Atlantic*, May 2013.

Sulmasy, Daniel. "Dignity and Bioethics: History, Theory, and Selected Applications." In *Human Dignity and Bioethics*, edited by Edmund D. Pellegrino, Adam Schulman, and Thomas W. Merrill, 469–501. Washington, DC: US Independent Agencies and Commissions, 2008.

———. "The Varieties of Human Dignity: A Logical and Conceptual Analysis." *Medicine, Health Care, and Philosophy* 16.4 (2013): 937–44.

Theixos, Heleana, and S. B. Jamil. "The Bad Habit of Bearing Children." *International Journal of Feminist Approaches to Bioethics* 7.1 (2014): 35–45.

Thomas, Dan. "Better Never to Have Been Born: Christian Ethics, Anti-abortion Politics, and the Pro-life Paradox." *Journal of Religious Ethics* 44.3 (2016): 518–42. doi:10.1111/jore.12152.

Thomson, Judith Jarvis. "A Defense of Abortion." *Philosophy and Public Affairs* 1.1 (1971): 47–66.

Tolkien, J. R. R. *The Letters of J. R. R. Tolkien.* Edited by Humphrey Carpenter. New York: Houghton Mifflin Harcourt, 2014.

Tollefsen, Christopher. "Response to Robert Koons and Matthew O'Brien's "Objects of Intention." *American Catholic Philosophical Quarterly* 87.4 (2013): 751–78.

Tooley, Michael. "Abortion and Infanticide." *Philosophy and Public Affairs* 2.1 (1972): 37–65.

US Conference of Catholic Bishops. *The Catholic Church in America: Meeting Real Needs in Your Neighborhood.* Washington, DC: Catholic Information Project, 2006.

Vaillant, George E. *Triumphs of Experience: The Men of the Harvard Grant Study.* Cambridge, MA: Harvard University Press, 2015.

Vanier, Jean. *From Brokenness to Community.* New York: Paulist Press, 1992.

Weaver, Janelle. "Social before Birth: Twins First Interact with Each Other as Fetuses: Twins Interact Purposefully in the Womb." *Scientific American,* January 1, 2011.

Wieland, Nellie. "Parental Obligation." *Utilitas* 23.3 (2011): 249–67.

Wiesel, Elisha. "Lessons from My Father: Elie Wiesel's Son on His Rebellion, and His Father's Love." *New York Jewish Week,* June 7, 2017. http://jewishweek .timesofisrael.com/lessons-from-my-father.

Wilcox, W. Bradford. *Why Marriage Matters: Thirty Conclusions from the Social Sciences.* 3rd ed. New York: Broadway Publications, 2011.

Witchel, Alex. "Father Rabbit." *New York Times,* November 22, 1992. www .nytimes.com/1992/11/22/style/father-rabbit.html?pagewanted=all.

Ye Hee Lee, Michelle. "Is the United States One of Seven Countries That 'Allow Elective Abortions after 20 Weeks of Pregnancy'?" *Washington Post,* October 9, 2017. https://www.washingtonpost.com/news/fact-checker/wp/2017/10/09 /is-the-united-states-one-of-seven-countries-that-allow-elective-abortions -after-20-weeks-of-pregnancy/?utm_term=.be069c8d50bd.

Index

adoption, 46–47, 63, 71, 93, 96–99
American Medical Association, 156,
  165–66
Aquinas, Thomas, Saint, 39, 56, 60, 103,
  115, 141, 183, 189
  apophatic theology, 11–12, 114
  limbo, 55
  persons, 4, 6
  Pauline Principle, 57
Aristotle, 172, 178
artificial gametes, 19–21, 25–26
artificial wombs, 61
artificially administered nutrition and
  hydration (ANH), 120
assisted suicide. *See* physician-assisted
  suicide
Augustine of Hippo, Saint, 55–56, 58,
  60, 102, 179
autonomy, 11, 17, 45, 140–41, 150
  bodily, 74
  dignity as reducible to, 122
  multiple meanings of, 129–30
  patient autonomy, 155, 157
  reproductive, 43
  suffering and, 131

basic rights, 4, 6, 20, 23, 32–35, 72, 76,
  85, 87, 124, 155
Bess, David, 109
Bovens, Luc, 135–39
Boyle, Joseph, 182
Brock, Stephen, 10, 182

capital punishment. *See* death penalty
Catholic tradition, 180
Chemerinsky, Erwin, 27–32, 39–41
claim right, 44–45
cloning, 19, 43, 45, 66
conjoined twins
  consent for surgery of, 186–90
  dignity of, 157, 178–80
  flourishing of, 187–80
  intentional killing of, 180–84
  marriage of, 188–89
  mutilation of, 184–86
conscience
  conscience clauses in law, 156, 166
  costs of abandoning, 164, 167–68
  diversity of medical profession, 164
  importance of for community, 163
  infanticide, 160
  respect for, 170, 172
consequentialist, 58
Cowden, Mhairi, 93–96
Cutas, Daniela, 21, 23–24

Davis, Michael, 32
death penalty, 33, 80–81, 90, 123, 154, 189
Declaration of Independence, 3, 146,
  155
Dell'Oro, Roberto, 171–73
dignity
  ambiguity of the term, 13, 15
  as attributed, 13, 121, 123–27
  as autonomy, 122, 129–32

dignity (*cont.*)
  as degreed quality, 14
  endowed, 121
  of every human being, ix, 6, 14, 32,
    35, 143, 147, 169, 171, 179
  as flourishing, 13, 120, 122–23
  as heuristic concept, 11
  as intrinsic, 13–18, 121, 127–29
Doss, Desmond T., 162–63, 168
double-effect reasoning, 173–74

ectogenesis, 61, 63, 65–66
ectopic pregnancy, 156, 183–84
  methotrexate (MXT), 183
Emanuel, E. J., 161–68
embryo adoption, 98
embryo experimentation, 20
embryo transfer (ET), 98
euthanasia
  definition of, 119
  dignity as attributed and, 123–27
  dignity as autonomy and, 129–32
  dignity as flourishing and, 122–23
  dignity as intrinsic worth and, 127–29
  weightiness argument against, 135–36
Evangelium Vitae (The Gospel of Life), 59
extrauterine pregnancy. *See* ectopic
  pregnancy

fallopian tube removal, 184
Fergusson, David M., 63
Feser, Edward, 37
fetal surgery, 87–95
Finnis, John, x, 44, 73, 80, 90, 132, 178,
  182
George, Robert, x, 31, 35, 127, 191
Gewirth, Alan, 17, 130
Girgis, Sherif, 14, 15
Giubilini, Alberto
  after-birth abortion, 40, 71–73,
    79–82, 86–91
  conscientious objection in health care,
    153–60
Goodwin, Michele, 27–32, 39–41
Gottman, John, 109
Grisez, Germain, x, 31, 182

Harris, John, 25–26
Hohfeld, Wesley, 44
Horwood, Karey, 97
Hughes, Glenn, 11
human action, 54, 137

in vitro fertilization (IVF), 22, 25, 30, 43

Jamil, S. B., 96–97
Jesus, 56, 59–60, 94, 102–3, 113–16
John Paul II, Pope
  on abortion, 58
  Evangelium vitae, 59
  on freedom of behavior, 175
  on freedom of conscience, 175
  Veritatis Splendor, 57

Kagan, Shelly, 1–3, 7–8
Kant, Immanuel, 6–7, 15, 127–30, 141,
  167
Kaveny, M. Cathleen, 185, 189–90
Keown, John, 132, 141
Kobylarz, Krzysztof, 178
Koons, Robert, 183

Leget, Carlo, 15–17
Levy, Neil, 76
Lewis, C. S., 103
Liao, S. Matthew, 93–95
liberty right, 44
Locke, John, 2, 72
Lotz, Mianna, 49–50
Lovering, Robert, 35–39

Macklin, Ruth, 122
Manninen, Bertha Alvarez, 72–76
Marquis, Don, 31, 33, 159
McMahan, Jeff, 80–81, 85, 90
methotrexate (MXT), 183
Minerva, Francesca, 40, 71–73, 79–82,
  86–91
mutilation, 177, 182, 184–85

Nelson, Thomas, 98–99
Neuhaus, Richard John, 56, 135
Newman, John Henry, 102, 111

O'Brien, Matthew, 183
organ donation, 40

Palacios-González, César, 25–26
parental duties, 47, 65
parental rights, 65
persistent vegetative state, 124
personal vocation, 102
personhood
    binary, nonscalar, 4, 14, 87
    lack of consensus about, 41
    Locke on, 72
    modal, 7
    threshold concept of, 87–88
physician-assisted suicide
    dignity as attributed and, 123–27
    dignity as autonomy and, 129–32
    dignity as flourishing and, 122–23
    dignity as intrinsic worth and,
        127–29
    financial burdens caused by, 146
    legal choice as burden, 144–46
    suicide contagion, 149
    undermining equality of persons,
        146–48
    undermining palliative care, 149–50
Porter, Lindsey, 78
Pruss, Alexander, 95–96, 103–4

Ranganathan, Bharat, 12–13
Räsänen, Joona
    defense of after-birth abortion, 79–91
    right to the death of the fetus, 61–69
reproductive autonomy, 43

revelation, 12, 180
Rini, Regina A., 77–78
Roe v. Wade, 27, 41, 156

Sartre, Jean-Paul, 114
Schuklenk, Udo, 139–42
Schwartz, Barry, 144
Singer, Peter, 1–3, 40
Smajdor, Anna, 21, 23–24
Sparrow, Robert, 48–49
Solzhenitsyn, Alexander, 104
speciesism
    capacity to suffer, 8–9
    definition of, 1
    moral intuition, 3
Stahl, R. Y., 161–68
Sulmasy, Daniel P., 13–15, 120–21, 127
surrogate motherhood, 19
Symposium (Plato), 94, 108

Testa, Giuseppe, 25–26
Theixos, Heleana, 96–97
Third Party Administrator (TPA), 169,
    171–75
Thomas, Dan, 53–60
Thomson, Judith Jarvis, 24, 80–81, 90,
    130
threshold view of personhood, 87–88, 90
Tooley, Michael, 17, 40, 72

van de Vathorst, Suzanne, 139–42
violinist argument, 24, 74, 80–81

Wieland, Nellie, 46-47

Christopher Kaczor

is professor of philosophy at Loyola Marymount University.
He is the author of a number of books, including *A Defense of Dignity:
Creating Life, Destroying Life, and Protecting the Rights of Conscience*
(University of Notre Dame Press, 2013).

Lightning Source UK Ltd.
Milton Keynes UK
UKHW021815210722
406195UK00008B/825